Communication Supports Checklist

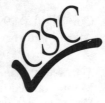

Communication Supports Checklist

For Programs Serving
Individuals with Severe Disabilities

A product of the National Joint Committee
for the Communication Needs of Persons with Severe Disabilities

by

Claire F. McCarthy, PT, M.S.   Lee K. McLean, Ph.D.

Jon F. Miller, Ph.D.   Diane Paul-Brown, Ph.D.

Mary Ann Romski, Ph.D.   Jane Davis Rourk, O.T.R./L.

David E. Yoder, Ph.D.

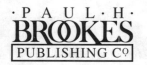

·P A U L·H·
BROOKES
PUBLISHING CO.

Baltimore • London • Toronto • Sydney

Paul H. Brookes Publishing Co.
Post Office Box 10624
Baltimore, Maryland 21285-0624

www.pbrookes.com

Typeset by Brushwood Graphics, Inc., Baltimore, Maryland.
Manufactured in the United States of America by
Versa Press, East Peoria, Illinois.

All royalties from the sale of this book will be used to further the work of the National Joint Committee for the Communication Needs of Persons with Severe Disabilities.

Most of the situations described in this book represent actual people and circumstances. Names have been changed to protect identities. Selected case studies are composites based on the authors' experiences; these case studies do not represent the lives or experiences of specific individuals, and no implications should be inferred. Case studies based on real programs or circumstances are presented herein with the programs' written consent.

Library of Congress Cataloging-in-Publication Data

Communication supports checklist for programs serving individuals with severe disabilities / Claire F. McCarthy . . . [et al.].
    p.   cm.
"A product of the National Joint Committee for the Communication Needs of Persons with Severe Disabilities."
Includes bibliographical references.
ISBN 1-55766-361-0
1. Handicapped—Means of communication—United States.   2. Speech-disorders—United States.   3. Communication devices for the disabled—United States.   4. Communication planning—United States.
I. McCarthy, Claire F., 1932–   .   II. National Joint Committee for the Communication Needs of Persons with Severe Disabilities (U.S.).
HV1569.4.C65   1998
362.4'048—dc21
                                                                                    98-24169
                                                                                    CIP

British Library Cataloguing in Publication data are available from the British Library.

Contents

Authors

Claire F. McCarthy, PT, M.S.
Director
Department of Physical Therapy and
    Occupational Therapy
Children's Hospital
300 Longwood Avenue
Boston, MA 02115

Lee K. McLean, Ph.D.
Director
A.J. Pappanikou Center
Professor
Department of Educational
    Psychology
University of Connecticut
249 Glenbrook Road, U-64
Storrs, CT 06269

Jon F. Miller, Ph.D.
Professor
Department of Communicative
    Disorders
University of Wisconsin–Madison
1975 Willow Drive
Madison, WI 53706

Diane Paul-Brown, Ph.D.
Director
Speech-Language Pathology
    Practices: Clinical Issues
American Speech-Language-Hearing
    Association
10801 Rockville Pike
Rockville, MD 20852

Mary Ann Romski, Ph.D.
Chair
National Joint Committee for the
    Communication Needs of Persons
    with Severe Disabilities
Professor
Departments of Communication,
    Psychology, and Educational
    Psychology & Special Education
Georgia State University
Atlanta, GA 30303

**Jane Davis Rourk, O.T.R./L., FAOTA,
    BCPOT**
Clinical Associate Professor
Division of Occupational Therapy
Department of Medical Allied Health
    Professions
University of North Carolina at
    Chapel Hill
CB #7335, Medical School Wing E
Chapel Hill, NC 27599

David E. Yoder, Ph.D.
Professor and Chair
Department of Medical Allied Health
    Professions
University of North Carolina at
    Chapel Hill
CB #7120, Medical School Wing E
Chapel Hill, NC 27599

Preface

Approximately 2 million Americans have severe communication disabilities, but there is a shortage of service providers who are prepared to address the communication needs of these people. In response to this need, the American Speech-Language-Hearing Association (ASHA) and The Association for Persons with Severe Handicaps (TASH) established the National Joint Committee for the Communication Needs of People with Severe Disabilities (NJC) in 1986 and invited other organizations to join.

The purpose of the NJC is to promote research, demonstration programs, and in-service/preservice education for service providers to help people with severe disabilities communicate effectively. As of 1998, member organizations included the American Association on Mental Retardation (AAMR); the American Occupational Therapy Association (AOTA); the American Physical Therapy Association (APTA); ASHA; the Council for Exceptional Children, Division for Children with Communication Disorders (CEC/DCCD); the United States Society for Augmentative and Alternative Communication (USSAAC); and TASH.

The NJC took as its first task amplification of the basic assumptions and recommendations reflected in the consensus statements issued by the Office of Special Education Programs (OSEP) and the TASH 1985 symposium. This amplification took the form of guidelines for meeting the communication needs of people with severe disabilities, including people with mental retardation requiring extensive to pervasive supports, autism, multiple disabilities, and other disorders (NJC, 1992).

The guidelines, which were endorsed by all member associations, included a Communication Bill of Rights (see p. 3) and three major program features to ensure these rights. These program features, critical to improving the communication skills of people with severe disabilities, include the following: 1) program support; 2) preferred practices in assessment, goal setting and intervention; and 3) interdisciplinary team knowledge and skills.

After a 1992 OSEP symposium on effective communication for children and youth with severe disabilities, the NJC recognized the need to translate its guidelines into a functional tool—a communication supports checklist that programs could use to improve communication supports and services for people with severe disabilities. Thus, the *Communication Supports Checklist for Programs Serving Individuals with Severe Disabilities* was developed by a subcommittee of NJC members: Claire F. McCarthy (APTA); Lee K. McLean (CEC/DCCD); Jon F. Miller (ASHA); Diane Paul-Brown (ASHA); Mary Ann Romski (AAMR), chair; Jane Davis Rourk (AOTA); and David E. Yoder (USSAAC).

The NJC thanks Kirsten Gardner, Vivian Lail-Davis, Jude Langsam, Mary Maxwell, Carolyn Stancliff, and Tawanna Tookes for their support during the preparation of this document. We are grateful to the programs that kindly completed the forms that appear as examples in this book. We also wish to thank the many people who reviewed this document at various stages of its evolution and assisted in the numerous revisions that led to the final product.

REFERENCE

National Joint Committee for the Communicative Needs of Persons with Severe Disabilities. (1992). Guidelines for meeting the communication needs of persons with severe disabilities. *Asha, 34*(Suppl. 7), 1–8.

The Importance of Communication

Rachel discusses her evening plans with her friend in the coffee area.

Jared sees his father pick up his car keys and walk toward the garage door. Jared makes a high-pitched vocalization and becomes very animated.

At a cocktail party, Diane glances at her wrist to indicate to her husband that it's time to leave.

Ahmad wheels up to the shopping mall information booth in his electric wheelchair and presses a button on a small talking computer to ask for directions to a jewelry store.

John, a fifth-grade student with mental retardation, points to a high shelf where his favorite book is located.

Jaspreet's new baby cries all night, and she and her husband try to determine if their child is wet, hungry, or sick.

Max and David each use pictures on their own communication boards to indicate that they want to go outside.

Mary and Yumiko use the TV menu on their picture communication boards to indicate which TV program they want to watch tonight.

Five people negotiate a student's goals and objectives in a team meeting.

Joaquin and his job coach are working on a new assembly task. Joaquin suddenly stands up, throws his materials on the floor, hits the side of his head with his fist, and runs screaming out of the room.

In her first-grade classroom, Susan turns to her classmate and points to the jar of finger paint. Her classmate opens the jar for her, and Susan begins to paint.

Two deaf friends laugh as one signs a joke to the other.

What do all these people have in common? They are all communicating. In these varied examples, we see some of the many different ways people communicate with each other. We use speech, signing, gestures, facial expressions, communication boards, and talking computers in various combinations to convey a range of information and feelings.

COMMUNICATION BILL OF RIGHTS

The ability to express feelings, interests, preferences, desires, and needs in some mode of communication is critical to the quality of life for all people. Recognizing the important role that communication plays in the quality of life is central to providing effective services and supports to people with severe disabilities. The access to communication that so many of us have *cannot* be taken for granted. A Communication Bill of Rights (see p. 3) helps remind us of just how extensive and important these privileges are. Although the rights listed may seem quite basic, it is quickly apparent just how meaningful they are; in addition, it is also readily apparent that these rights are often unavailable or are even denied to people for whom communicating is difficult.

All too often, people with severe disabilities encounter significant difficulty communicating with the people in their lives. Many people with severe disabilities communicate in nonconventional ways, use nonspeech systems for communication, or produce speech that may be difficult to understand. Since the early 1980s, we have seen remarkable advances in our knowledge of how communication develops and how we use communication. These advances have allowed us to design more meaningful assessments, more appropriate intervention plans, and more supportive communication environments for people with severe disabilities. Since the mid-1990s, there have been major improvements in our ability to provide augmentative and alternative and communication (AAC) modes that allow people who do not speak to communicate more effectively. Such AAC improvements include digitized and synthesized speech output, word prediction capabilities, and expanded user-access options (e.g., gaze, voice recognition). Although we cannot yet solve all of the communication challenges faced by people with severe disabilities, these developments should allow us to make great improvements in our communication supports and services for children and adults with severe disabilities.

KNOWLEDGE–PRACTICE GAP

Unfortunately, the gap between our knowledge and our practice regarding communication is still significant. This gap was a central theme and point of discussion at a 1992 national symposium on effective communication for children and youth with severe disabilities sponsored by the U.S. Department of Education. At this symposium, one keynote speaker commented,

> We have a dream about a social environment that encourages and enables communication with individuals with severe disabilities. . . . [To achieve this dream, it] is not enough for us to teach the skills necessary for communication to individuals with disabilities; we must also create an environment in which there will be people who desire, and know how, to interact with any person, regardless of that person's level of function. . . . We cannot merely talk about how important it is to provide effective communication systems for all persons, we must devise a plan to make it happen. (Yoder, 1992, p. 302)

Another speaker at the same symposium noted,

> We should all realize . . . that our philosophical holdings and our revised language do not themselves specify how we will attain our values and our educational goals. . . . Too often, I see inclusionary school settings that really don't include, parent involvement that intimidates rather than involves, and the teaching of functional communication skills that would never be used or be useful in real world interactions. . . . The translation of our words into action demands a rigor, a commitment of resources, and a willingness to totally re-engineer our educational contexts [not] adequately reflected in most of the educational settings with which I am familiar. (McLean, 1993, pp. 1–2)

Communication Bill of Rights

All people with a disability of any extent or severity have a basic right to affect, through communication, the conditions of their existence. All people have the following specific communication rights in their daily interactions. These rights are summarized from the Communication Bill of Rights put forth in 1992 by the National Joint Committee for the Communication Needs of Persons with Severe Disabilities.

Each person has the right to:

✓ Request desired objects, actions, events, and people

✓ Refuse undesired objects, actions, or events

✓ Express personal preferences and feelings

✓ Be offered choices and alternatives

✓ Reject offered choices

✓ Request and receive another person's attention and interaction

✓ Ask for and receive information about changes in routine and environment

✓ Receive intervention to improve communication skills

✓ Receive a response to any communication, whether or not the responder can fulfill the request

✓ Have access to AAC (augmentative and alternative communication) and other AT (assistive technology) services and devices at all times

✓ Have AAC and other AT devices that function properly at all times

✓ Be in environments that promote one's communication as a full partner with other people, including peers

✓ Be spoken to with respect and courtesy

✓ Be spoken to directly and not be spoken for or talked about in the third person while present

✓ Have clear, meaningful, and culturally and linguistically appropriate communications

From the National Joint Committee for the Communicative Needs of Persons with Severe Disabilities. (1992). Guidelines for meeting the communication needs of persons with severe disabilities. *Asha, 34*(Suppl. 7), 2–3; adapted by permission.

In today's world of managed care, with its emphasis on the "bottom line," the challenge of providing communication supports and services that reflect what we now consider to be recommended practices is greater than ever. The return on health care dollars invested in services for people with severe disabilities is maximized in programs that adopt such practices. If we are to close the gap between our knowledge and our practices, this effort must come from the families and service providers who support individuals with severe disabilities. For this reason, the National Joint Committee for the Communication Needs of Persons with Severe Disabilities has designed the *Communication Supports Checklist for Programs Serving Individuals with Severe Disabilities* (CSC) to enable your team to identify the gaps in your own service settings and begin closing those gaps.

IMPROVING PROGRAM SUPPORT FOR COMMUNICATION

There are many ways that program settings and practices can support communication for all people. This checklist is designed to help your team look at your program systematically and address the following questions:

- Do our practices support and respect the communication rights of the individuals we serve?
- Do our settings support and promote meaningful communication in natural contexts?
- Do our assessment, goal-setting, and program implementation practices conform to current recommended practices?
- Does our team have the knowledge and skills needed to support the communication needs of people with severe disabilities?

In the pages that follow, you will be introduced to the Communication Supports Checklist, a flexible instrument that allows you to assess your program's strengths and weaknesses. You can then develop a Communication Supports Action Plan to build on these strengths and simultaneously work on areas identified for improvement. This Action Plan will help you to better serve all people with severe communication disabilities in your program. A flowchart (see Figure 1) illustrates the Checklist process and the subsequent development of an Action Plan.

To help guide you through this program assessment and action-planning process, we provide Checklist and Action Plan forms that have been completed by two separate teams. The first team is from a school in a large metropolitan area on the East Coast; the second team is based in a semirural area in a southeastern state. The two teams' completed forms are located after the blank Checklist and Action Plan forms and are followed by a glossary of terms that are mentioned throughout the book.

REFERENCES

McLean, L. (1993). Assuring best practices in communication for children and youth with severe disabilities. *Clinics in Communication Disorders, 3*(2), 1–6.

National Joint Committee for the Communicative Needs of Persons with Severe Disabilities. (1992). Guidelines for meeting the communication needs of persons with severe disabilities. *Asha, 34*(Suppl. 7), 1–8.

Yoder, D.E. (1992). Dreams, schemes, teams, flying machines, and persons with severe communication disabilities. In L. Küpper (Ed.), *The second national symposium on effective communication for children and youth with severe disabilities: Topic papers, reader's guide, and videotape* (pp. 301–306). McLean, VA: Interstate Research Associates.

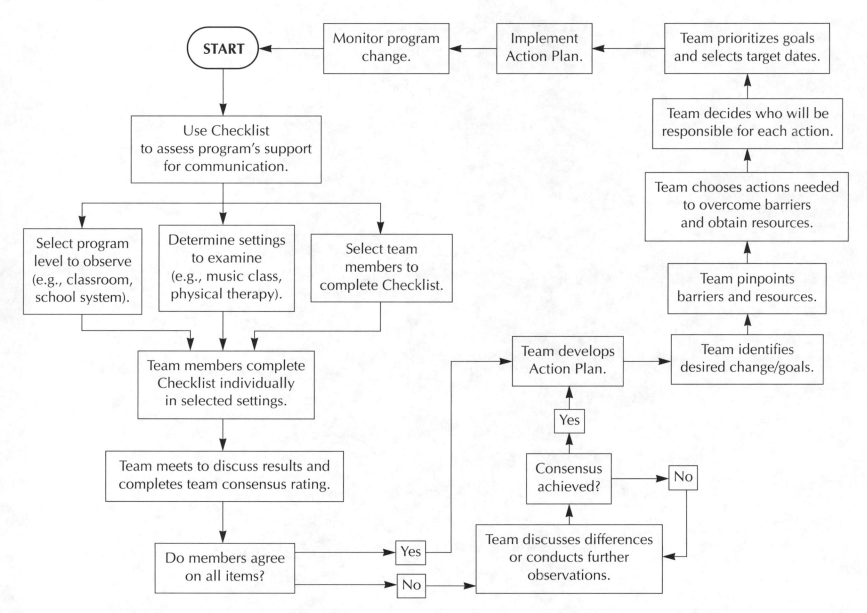

Figure 1. Using the Communication Supports Checklist and Action Plan.

How to Use the Communication Supports Checklist

The Checklist has been designed to help your team develop a shared understanding and vision for your program. The very process of completing the Checklist together will provide a valuable opportunity for you to discuss and compare your individual perspectives, values, and beliefs about the communication supports and services provided by your program. As you rate the Checklist items, you may find that you are looking at your program's settings and practices in new ways. You may find that team members have very different perspectives and experiences, even though you all work with individuals in the same program. You will certainly discover that, in many ways, your team is already doing many things that reflect recommended practices. It is also likely that you will find some areas needing improvement that you had not considered before.

COMPONENTS OF THE CHECKLIST

The Checklist contains 97 items and is divided into three major sections:

1. Overall Program Support for Communication
2. Assessment Practices, Goal-Setting Practices, and Program Implementation
3. Team Competencies

The items in the first section, Overall Program Support for Communication, address your program's values, attitudes, and beliefs about people with communication disabilities. The second section, Assessment Practices, Goal-Setting Practices, and Program Implementation, will help you determine the comprehensiveness and adequacy of the communication services and supports that are being provided for individuals in your program. The third section, Team Competencies, will permit you to determine the collective knowledge and skills that team members bring to your program. Familiarize yourself with all items in each section before team members complete the Checklist individually. Determine which Checklist items apply to your program. For example, if no individuals in a supported living program take medication, that program's team may want to skip Item 76 (see p. 35).

WHERE AND WHEN TO USE THE CHECKLIST

The Checklist is designed so that it is you who decides the level of administration (e.g., individual classroom, total school system) as well as the frequency of administration (e.g., annual, biannual). The Checklist can be used to inventory the communication characteristics of just one environment within a program or of an entire program. The choice is yours. For example, you might want to inventory the communication supports in an English class that includes one student with a severe disability, or you might choose to look at communication supports throughout an entire school system. Similarly, your focus may be just one family's home or an entire residential program. The emphasis of the CSC is on the program. Therefore, the Checklist is not intended to assess an individual's communication skills; rather, it concentrates on how a program supports the communication of all individuals served by the program. At a minimum, the program should be reevaluated annually using the Checklist, but reevaluation should occur more frequently if the team decides that this is appropriate.

WHO SHOULD COMPLETE THE CHECKLIST

We suggest that interdisciplinary teams use the Checklist. Above all, the team completing the Checklist should include the individual or individuals who are supported by the program and/or their family members or advocates. The team may need to make special accommodations (e.g., adjusting positioning, providing communication devices) to ensure that the individuals supported by the program can provide input when completing the Checklist. Depending on the nature of the environment, the team might also include friends, administrators, audiologists, occupational therapists, ophthalmolo-gists, physical therapists, physicians or nurse-practitioners, psychologists, rehabilitation engineers, special educators, speech-language pathologists, support personnel, teachers, and others who interact regularly with the individual or individuals in the environment being inventoried.

INSTRUCTIONS FOR COMPLETING THE CHECKLIST

Before you begin, make a copy of the Checklist for each person on your team. You may also want to distribute copies of the Glossary (see p. 211) to the members of the team if you think that this will reduce the amount of valuable meeting time spent explaining unfamiliar terms. Then, be sure to complete the descriptive information on the front page of the Checklist. Note whether the form is being used for an individual member rating or for the team consensus rating, and write down the specific focus of the self-assessment (e.g., one classroom, an entire service agency). Fill in the date and names and roles/disciplines (e.g., individual served by program, physical therapist, parent) of the participating team members.

For each of the three sections of the Checklist, place a checkmark in the box that corresponds with one of these three descriptions:

- **Consistently True**
- **Sometimes True**
- **Rarely True**

A rating of **Consistently True** reflects your judgment that the item is uniformly and consistently true of the program. A rating of **Sometimes True** suggests that the program is doing well regarding the item but still needs improvement. A rating of **Rarely True** indicates that you believe the program rarely or never demonstrates that communication characteristic. Use the comment space to explain items rated **Sometimes**

True or **Rarely True,** and add any other comments that you think will help when your team reviews these ratings, completes the team consensus rating, and develops an Action Plan.

Remember that these ratings are for your use in assessing your program's relative strengths and areas of needed improvement. Thus, the ratings assigned give a concrete measure to help you plan and monitor your program's improvement efforts. For the CSC to serve its purpose, team members must feel free to assign ratings that reflect their personal opinions and experiences about current program policies, practices, and expertise. To ensure that team members can openly and freely participate, these ratings *must not* be used as scores by agencies or administrators for external evaluation of any program!

INDIVIDUAL MEMBER RATING

Typically, each team member should complete all three sections of the Checklist independently, based on his or her knowledge and experiences in the program. Individual team members may evaluate different settings (e.g., classroom, gym, worksite) or may choose to focus on just one section or on selected items of the Checklist.

TEAM CONSENSUS RATING

Following the completion of each team member's ratings, the team should come together for two to four team meetings, scheduled as closely together as possible, to discuss the results of the individual member ratings and to complete a new Checklist, which will serve as the team consensus rating. Before the first meeting, make another copy of the Checklist from this book, and check the team consensus rating box on the cover sheet. Fill in the names and roles/disciplines of the participating team members. During each meeting, the team should work toward consensus so a meaningful Action Plan can be developed to improve and maintain communication supports in the program.

As your team reaches consensus on each item, record your team rating and any explanatory comments on the team consensus rating form. When there are significant differences of opinion in any area, additional program observations or discussion will be necessary.

✓✓✓

There is disagreement among members of one school's team about Checklist Item 19 (see p. 18). The speech-language pathologist has checked Consistently True because he assumes that all the students with severe disabilities in the program have their augmentative and alternative communication (AAC) devices with them in all academic settings. The physical therapist, however, has yet to observe AAC devices being brought along when two of the three students with severe disabilities in the program attend physical therapy sessions. At this point, the paraprofessional explains that the devices are taken from the students during recess for "safekeeping." After discussion, the team agrees that the most accurate rating at this time is Rarely True.

PHOTOCOPYING RELEASE

You may photocopy any part of the *Communication Supports Checklist for Programs Serving Individuals with Severe Disabilities* for distribution for program and staff development and educational purposes. Although photocopying for such purposes is unlimited, no part of the book may be reproduced to generate revenue for any program or individual. Photocopies must be made from an original book.

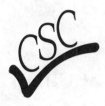

Communication Supports Checklist

For Programs Serving Individuals with Severe Disabilities

Check one: ☐ Individual member rating   ☐ Team consensus rating

Program(s) and/or setting(s) evaluated: Date:

_____   _____

_____   _____

_____   _____

_____   _____

Checklist completed by (list individual rater or team members and their roles/disciplines):

_____   _____

_____   _____

_____   _____

_____   _____

Communication Supports Checklist • McCarthy et al. • © 1998 Paul H. Brookes Publishing Co., Inc., Baltimore

Section I

Overall Program Support for Communication

Instructions for Rating Items in this Section

When evaluating the program's Overall Program Support for Communication, your team should consider how much program policies, decisions, and practices reflect the values, attitudes, and beliefs listed in Parts A, B, and C of this section. Consider the program's written policies and routine practices as you evaluate these items. A rating of **Consistently True** means that this indicator is true of the attitudes and practices of virtually everyone who interacts with individuals served by the program. A rating of **Sometimes True** should be assigned if you feel that many (but not all) of the staff practices and agency policies are consistent with the attitude or belief identified in an item. A rating of **Rarely True** indicates that a particular attitude or value is rarely or never reflected in the program's routine policies and practices with individuals who have severe disabilities.

A. Philosophy

The following values, attitudes, and beliefs about communication are desirable in all decisions and interactions with individuals with severe disabilities. As a team, we behave in ways that reflect these beliefs:

	Consistently True	Sometimes True	Rarely True	COMMENTS
1. Communication is a basic human right.				
2. All individuals should have opportunities to participate fully in their community.				
3. All individuals should have freedom of action and choice.				
4. All individuals communicate in some way; communication may be nonspoken, nonsymbolic, and/or nonintentional.				

Communication Supports Checklist • McCarthy et al. • © 1998 Paul H. Brookes Publishing Co., Inc., Baltimore

A.   Philosophy

(continued)

The following values, attitudes, and beliefs about communication are desirable in all decisions and interactions with individuals with severe disabilities. As a team, we behave in ways that reflect these beliefs:	Consistently True	Sometimes True	Rarely True	COMMENTS
5. Appropriate communication goals improve quality of life.				
6. Individuals with severe disabilities and their primary communication partners are involved in communication goal setting and intervention.				
7. Individual and family choices are respected.				
8. Diverse family values and traditions are recognized and respected.				

A.   Philosophy   *(continued)*

The following values, attitudes, and beliefs about communication are desirable in all decisions and interactions with individuals with severe disabilities. As a team, we behave in ways that reflect these beliefs:	Consistently True	Sometimes True	Rarely True	COMMENTS
9. Team collaboration is essential for effective service.				

Communication Supports Checklist • McCarthy et al. • © 1998 Paul H. Brookes Publishing Co., Inc., Baltimore

B.   Protection of Communication Rights

CSC ✓

The program ensures the basic communication rights of individuals, regardless of the nature or severity of their disabilities. In the settings being inventoried, communication partners:	Consistently True	Sometimes True	Rarely True	COMMENTS
10. Recognize and acknowledge initiations for social interactions.				
11. Recognize and acknowledge requests (for objects, actions, events, people, information, and feedback).				
12. Recognize and acknowledge expressions of feelings and attitudes.				
13. Honor preferences indicated by individuals.				

Communication Supports Checklist • McCarthy et al. • © 1998 Paul H. Brookes Publishing Co., Inc., Baltimore

B.   Protection of Communication Rights   *(continued)*

The program ensures the basic communication rights of individuals, regardless of the nature or severity of their disabilities. In the settings being inventoried, communication partners:	Consistently True	Sometimes True	Rarely True	COMMENTS
14. Offer multiple choices in activities throughout the day.				
15. Acknowledge and honor rejections unless the undesired action, event, or object is essential to the individual's protection from harm.				
16. Arrange comprehensive communication assessments and individually appropriate interventions for individuals who might benefit from communication intervention services, regardless of age and severity of disability.				
17. Include peers without disabilities who convey respect and courtesy.				

B. Protection of Communication Rights (continued)

The program ensures the basic communication rights of individuals, regardless of the nature or severity of their disabilities. In the settings being inventoried, communication partners:	Consistently True	Sometimes True	Rarely True	COMMENTS
18. Do not discuss an individual in the third person when that individual is present.				
19. Ensure that individuals have access to assistive technology (AT), augmentative and alternative communication (AAC) devices, and support systems needed for communication at all times.				
20. Ensure that AT and AAC devices are in good working order at all times.				
21. Offer information and explanations when appropriate (e.g., introductions to a classroom or jobsite visitor, explanation about the need to change a planned activity).				

C. Environmental Support for Communication

The environments in which people learn, live, play, and work should promote and support communication. People in each of our program's settings do so by:	Consistently True	Sometimes True	Rarely True	COMMENTS
22. Expecting communication (e.g., waiting for an initiation or a response, maintaining visual contact).				
23. Providing interesting and age-appropriate materials, communication partners, and activities.				
24. Following policies and practices that do not prohibit or restrict communication.				
25. Including communication partners who know how to use AAC systems and devices used by individuals (e.g., American Sign Language, graphic symbols, high- and low-technology devices).				

C. Environmental Support for Communication (continued)

The environments in which people learn, live, play, and work should promote and support communication. People in each of our program's settings do so by:	Consistently True	Sometimes True	Rarely True		COMMENTS
26. Arranging materials so individuals without symbolic communication skills can indicate their interests or requests through the use of gaze, natural gestures, and/or vocal or behavioral signals.					
27. Including peers without disabilities who are available for communication interactions.					
28. Including communication partners who use appropriate language (e.g., primary language) and appropriate communication mode(s) (e.g., oral, signed, graphic, adapted for vision or hearing impairments).					

Communication Supports Checklist • McCarthy et al. • © 1998 Paul H. Brookes Publishing Co., Inc., Baltimore

Section II

Assessment Practices, Goal-Setting Practices, and Program Implementation

Instructions for Rating Items in this Section

When evaluating the program's Assessment Practices, Goal-Setting Practices, and Program Implementation, your team should consider whether and how much the program's actual practices are consistent with the ideal practices identified in Parts A, B, and C of this section. Consider the program's written procedural policies and routine practices as you consider these items. When rating each item, a rating of **Consistently True** means the statement is consistently true of the practices used by all people involved in communication assessment, goal setting, and program implementation. A rating of **Sometimes True** might indicate some efforts to adopt the practices in the program or that one or two staff members in the program do use the practices. A rating of **Rarely True** indicates that a particular practice is rarely or never reflected in the way that communication needs and abilities are assessed, the way that goals are established, and/or the way that a program is implemented for individuals with severe disabilities served by your program.

A. Assessment Practices

Communication interactions should be observed carefully before program implementation is designed. The degree to which settings are sensitive and responsive to each person's communication needs should also be observed. Goals can be chosen for individuals and the places where they learn, live, play, and work. When assessing an individual's communication abilities and needs, team members:	Consistently True	Sometimes True	Rarely True	COMMENTS
29. Describe the individual's current communication modes (including intentional, nonintentional, symbolic, and non-symbolic communication).				
30. Include measures of sensory responsivity (i.e., hearing and vision tests) by appropriate professionals.				
31. Include measures of physical status (e.g., positioning, sensorimotor, joint range of motion, motor control) by appropriate professionals.				
32. Identify social functions (e.g., comment, protest, request) of communication behavior across settings.				

A. Assessment Practices

(continued)

Communication interactions should be observed carefully before program implementation is designed. The degree to which settings are sensitive and responsive to each person's communication needs should also be observed. Goals can be chosen for individuals and the places where they learn, live, play, and work. When assessing an individual's communication abilities and needs, team members:

	Consistently True	Sometimes True	Rarely True	COMMENTS
33. Identify the individual's primary communication partners.				
34. Conduct multiple observations over time.				
35. Measure the responsiveness of partners to communication acts.				
36. Measure opportunities for communication across environments (e.g., education, living, leisure, work).				

Communication Supports Checklist • McCarthy et al. • © 1998 Paul H. Brookes Publishing Co., Inc., Baltimore

A.   Assessment Practices

(continued)

Communication interactions should be observed carefully before program implementation is designed. The degree to which settings are sensitive and responsive to each person's communication needs should also be observed. Goals can be chosen for individuals and the places where they learn, live, play, and work. When assessing an individual's communication abilities and needs, team members:

	Consistently True	Sometimes True	Rarely True	COMMENTS
37. Identify the specific communication forms and uses in various modes (e.g., speech, writing, AAC) that are useful across settings.				
38. Measure the spontaneity of communication.				
39. Use a team model that includes the individual, family members, peers, friends, professionals, support personnel, and other significant communication partners.				
40. Specifically ask family members to provide information about perceived communication needs.				

A. Assessment Practices

Communication interactions should be observed carefully before program implementation is designed. The degree to which settings are sensitive and responsive to each person's communication needs should also be observed. Goals can be chosen for individuals and the places where they learn, live, play, and work. When assessing an individual's communication abilities and needs, team members:

	Consistently True	Sometimes True	Rarely True	COMMENTS
41. Provide explanations of assessment procedures and results in ways that are meaningful to all team members, including the individual with severe disabilities.				
42. Provide information about communication needs that partners notice during their activities and interactions with individuals.				

B. Goal-Setting Practices

When reaching consensus on appropriate and attainable program implementation goals for an individual, the team:	Consistently True	Sometimes True	Rarely True	COMMENTS
43. Selects and prioritizes goals based on their importance and potential impact on an individual's quality of life.				
44. Uses a team model that includes the individual as well as family members, peers, friends, professionals, support personnel, and other significant communication partners during the planning and implementation of communication interventions.				
45. Considers environmental as well as individual goals.				
46. Takes into account an individual's existing intentional (e.g., pointing to a picture display) and/or nonintentional (e.g., crying) communication abilities.				

B. Goal-Setting Practices

When reaching consensus on appropriate and attainable program implementation goals for an individual, the team:	Consistently True	Sometimes True	Rarely True	COMMENTS
47. Selects goals consistent with a logical hierarchy of skills and identifies short-term objectives that seem realistically attainable for an individual within a specified time frame (e.g., 6 months, 1 year).				
48. Selects short-term objectives that are consistent with the long-term goals for an individual.				
49. Selects goals that will support an individual's transition to a new environment (e.g., from school to work).				
50. Reviews information from previous teams to ensure continuity of an individual's goals (e.g., person worked on two-choice picture-pointing skills in previous program as a step toward use of a more complex communication board. In new program, team agrees to move on to three-choice picture board).				

C.   Program Implementation

Program implementation is based on assessment and selected functional communication goals across settings. Ongoing evaluation is used to measure outcomes and adjust practices accordingly. When implementing intervention programs, the team:

	Consistently True	Sometimes True	Rarely True	COMMENTS
51. Targets communication goals primarily in an individual's natural environments during typical interactions, rather than in isolated environments.				
52. Uses pull-out intervention only when necessary for additional practice.				
53. Provides opportunities for initiation, maintenance, and termination of communication/social interactions.				
54. Provides opportunities to communicate across all environments.				

Communication Supports Checklist • McCarthy et al. • © 1998 Paul H. Brookes Publishing Co., Inc., Baltimore

C. Program Implementation

Program implementation is based on assessment and selected functional communication goals across settings. Ongoing evaluation is used to measure outcomes and adjust practices accordingly. When implementing intervention programs, the team:	Consistently True	Sometimes True	Rarely True	COMMENTS
55. Uses an individual's current communication systems while promoting new skill acquisition.				
56. Uses communication supports and systems that are appropriate to each individual's physical abilities.				
57. Uses communication supports and systems that are appropriate to each individual's sensory abilities.				
58. Uses communication supports and systems that are appropriate to each individual's cognitive abilities.				

C. Program Implementation

Program implementation is based on assessment and selected functional communication goals across settings. Ongoing evaluation is used to measure outcomes and adjust practices accordingly. When implementing intervention programs, the team:

	Consistently True	Sometimes True	Rarely True	COMMENTS
59. Uses communication supports and systems that are appropriate to each individual's communication needs and environments across settings.				
60. Includes necessary adaptations or modifications to the environment to optimize an individual's use of communication supports and systems (e.g., mounting AAC device on wheelchair).				
61. Provides for the seating and positioning needs of individuals who use communication supports and systems.				
62. Makes assistive devices available to help individuals use supports for communication (e.g., hand/wrist splint, head-controlled pointer, control switches).				

C. Program Implementation

(continued)

Program implementation is based on assessment and selected functional communication goals across settings. Ongoing evaluation is used to measure outcomes and adjust practices accordingly. When implementing intervention programs, the team:

	Consistently True	Sometimes True	Rarely True	COMMENTS
63. Integrates elements of individual instruction by all team members involved.				
64. Implements plans as designed to accomplish stated goals.				
65. Uses a team model that includes the individual, family members, friends, peers, professionals, support personnel, and other significant communication partners.				
66. Builds on goals and strategies developed in previous programs.				

Communication Supports Checklist • McCarthy et al. • © 1998 Paul H. Brookes Publishing Co., Inc., Baltimore

C.   Program Implementation

Program implementation is based on assessment and selected functional communication goals across settings. Ongoing evaluation is used to measure outcomes and adjust practices accordingly. When implementing intervention programs, the team:	Consistently True	Sometimes True	Rarely True	COMMENTS
67. Includes and implements plans for continuity and transfer of information regarding communication supports and services before an individual changes program placement.				
68. Includes a specific time schedule for team reassessment of all program elements.				

Communication Supports Checklist • McCarthy et al. • © 1998 Paul H. Brookes Publishing Co., Inc., Baltimore

Section III

Team Competencies

Instructions for Rating Items in this Section

Rate the knowledge and skills that team members contribute as combined resources. Specific types of knowledge and skills are identified in Parts A and B of this section. Consider the specific training, experiences, and expertise of each team member, including family members, as you consider these items. When rating these items, a rating of **Consistently True** means that one or more team members has outstanding knowledge, skills, and/or experience relevant to that particular item. A rating of **Sometimes True** should be assigned if you believe that one or two (but not all) team members demonstrate this knowledge or skill. A rating of **Sometimes True** should also be assigned if you have the occasional help of a resource person (not a regular member of the team), but the team agrees that it would be desirable for additional team members to share this knowledge or skill or that the levels of expertise could be improved. A rating of **Rarely True** indicates that a particular knowledge or skill is clearly not demonstrated by any single member of the team.

A.   Knowledge

Collectively, the team's knowledge supports and encourages communication. At least one team member has knowledge about:	Consistently True	Sometimes True	Rarely True	COMMENTS
69. Human development.				
70. Communication development, including reading and writing.				
71. Individuals with severe disabilities across ages and levels of independence.				
72. Factors that prevent secondary conditions that interfere with communication (e.g., swallowing disorders, poor positioning, challenging behavior).				

A. Knowledge

(continued)

Collectively, the team's knowledge supports and encourages communication. At least one team member has knowledge about:	Consistently True	Sometimes True	Rarely True	COMMENTS
73. Different means of communication (e.g., body posture, vocalization, gaze, gesture, sign language, electronic and nonelectronic systems).				
74. Different types of communication symbols (e.g., pictures, braille, words, signs, speech).				
75. Amplification and other AT useful to people who have severe disabilities with accompanying sensory limitations.				
76. Medications and their effects on behavior, especially communication.				

A.   Knowledge

Collectively, the team's knowledge supports and encourages communication. At least one team member has knowledge about:	Consistently True	Sometimes True	Rarely True	COMMENTS
77. Motor control, muscle tone, and positioning as these affect communication.				
78. Disabilities that may co-occur with communication disorders (e.g., feeding and swallowing problems, seizures, sensory impairments).				
79. Challenging behavior as a potential communication act.				
80. Designing and working with a variety of service delivery models (e.g., classroom-based, pull-out, collaborative).				

A. Knowledge

(continued)

Collectively, the team's knowledge supports and encourages communication. At least one team member has knowledge about:	Consistently True	Sometimes True	Rarely True	COMMENTS
81. Family dynamics and the impact of severe disability on the family.				
82. The importance of incorporating current research findings into assessment and program implementation.				

Communication Supports Checklist • McCarthy et al. • © 1998 Paul H. Brookes Publishing Co., Inc., Baltimore

B.   Skills and Experience

Team members' skills, experiences, and access to resources support and encourage communication. At least one team member has demonstrated the expertise or has the help of resource people who know how to:	Consistently True	Sometimes True	Rarely True	COMMENTS
83. Integrate the domains of cognitive, motor, sensory, and social functioning in communication *assessment* and *goal setting*.				
84. Integrate the domains of cognitive, motor, sensory, and social functioning in communication *implementation*.				
85. Provide ongoing assessment and evaluation using standardized and nonstandardized (formal or informal) procedures.				
86. Plan and implement communication assessments that lead directly to functional communication intervention goals and objectives.				

Communication Supports Checklist • McCarthy et al. • © 1998 Paul H. Brookes Publishing Co., Inc., Baltimore

B. Skills and Experience

(continued)

Team members' skills, experiences, and access to resources support and encourage communication. At least one team member has demonstrated the expertise or has the help of resource people who know how to:	Consistently True	Sometimes True	Rarely True	COMMENTS
87. Describe and document functional communication abilities and needs within specific contexts (e.g., educational settings, living environments, recreational environments, vocational environments, the community at large).				
88. Plan, implement, monitor, and modify, as needed, intervention programs that allow individuals to develop functional communication skills in spoken or AAC modes appropriate to educational, living, recreational, and work environments.				
89. Assess emergent and functional literacy skills across all environments.				
90. Teach emergent and functional literacy skills across all environments.				

B. Skills and Experience

Team members' skills, experiences, and access to resources support and encourage communication. At least one team member has demonstrated the expertise or has the help of resource people who know how to:	Consistently True	Sometimes True	Rarely True	COMMENTS
91. Help the individual use the most appropriate (and least intrusive) positioning and mobility aids to maximize functional communication across a variety of environments.				
92. Manage activities of daily living and incorporate functional communication into each of these activities.				
93. Integrate cognition; oral and written communication; and motor, sensory, and social development in defining and implementing communication goals.				
94. Incorporate current research findings into assessment and program implementation.				

B.   Skills and Experience

Team members' skills, experiences, and access to resources support and encourage communication. At least one team member has demonstrated the expertise or has the help of resource people who know how to:

	Consistently True	Sometimes True	Rarely True	COMMENTS
95. Promote team participation and self-advocacy on the part of individuals with severe disabilities.				
96. Interact in a culturally sensitive manner.				
97. Understand laws that protect the rights of people with severe disabilities.				

How to Develop Your Communication Supports Action Plan

After completing your team consensus rating form, use the results to develop an Action Plan for improving any aspect(s) of the program that you identified as needing improvement.

COMPONENTS OF THE ACTION PLAN

The Action Plan form contains the same items as the Checklist and is divided into the same three parts (Overall Program Support for Communication; Assessment Practices, Goal-Setting Practices, and Program Implementation; and Team Competencies). To help your team structure its action-planning process, the Action Plan form is divided into six columns:

1. Desired Change/Goals
2. Barriers and Resources
3. Action Needed
4. Who
5. Priority
6. When

We suggest that you complete the first four columns for all items in the Action Plan before you complete the last two columns (Priority and When). Do not feel restricted to the space allotted on the form.

✓✓✓

When one team completed the team consensus rating, it identified a concern in Checklist Item 14 related to providing adequate choices across all daily activities (see p. 17). Team members realized that choices were rarely offered outside meals, and the options offered were usually either/or choices only (e.g., "Do you want cheese or peanut butter?"). The team decided that a desired change would be "to increase options and opportunities for choice across a variety of activities."

Desired Change/Goals

The first issue for your team to consider, relative to each aspect of the program that is being reviewed, is whether your

Checklist led you to identify some practice or policy that you want to change or to improve. You might not feel a need to make changes to many of these items. If your team identifies a need for improvement, then try to state this need in terms of a concrete goal. Record this goal in the first column, Desired Change/Goals.

Barriers and Resources

When your team identifies a desired change, consider what steps need to be taken to achieve this change. Are there *barriers*—either within your agency or external to it—that must be addressed before change is possible? Such barriers could include state funding policies, attitudes of agency personnel or family members, lack of staff knowledge or expertise about communication, and so forth. To achieve your identified goals, do you need specific *resources*, such as designated planning time, funds for AAC devices, positioning equipment, and so forth? Unfortunately, there are often numerous barriers to goal achievement and/or few resources available. As you identify existing barriers and resources needed, record them in the Barriers and Resources column.

—————————————————————————— ✓✓✓

Members of the team that wanted to increase the number of offered choices identified two barriers. Some team members stated that they could not think of any way to include choices in their activities because they had never done this before. In addition, the physical therapist noted that the individuals really could not have a choice about participating in medically necessary activities. The team also recognized the need for additional information through training and/or technical assistance to overcome the barriers that it identified.

—————————————————————————————

Action Needed

Once you have identified specific barriers to achieving your team's program improvement goals, the next step is to identify the specific actions that you can take, as team members, to overcome the identified barriers and gain access to needed resources. These actions may include conducting in-service training for other program staff on how to recognize and respond to nonsymbolic communication, meeting with agency administrators, and contacting your state's assistive technology resource center. Your team should concentrate on very specific actions that it can actually carry out.

—————————————————————————— ✓✓✓

The team that identified a lack of experience in designing opportunities for choice as one barrier to its goals identified two actions needed to overcome the barrier. The Action Plan stated that the team would schedule time with a member of the agency's staff or an outside consultant to help team members figure out how to incorporate at least three opportunities for choice in their activities. The Action Plan also stated that the team would try to increase the number of choices within each opportunity.

—————————————————————————————

For instance, if you identified a critical resource that is available only to an upper-level administrator who is not participating in this program review and action-planning process, then your immediate action might be to schedule a meeting with this administrator to explain your needs and present your specific request.

Who

In the fourth column of the Action Plan form, record the initials of the specific team member(s) who agree to be responsible for each identified action. Even though all team members may agree to participate in or to assist with a particular activity, designate one or two individuals as having the primary responsibility for initiating this action and monitoring its accomplishment. For example, the speech-language pathologist on the team that wanted to increase offered choices agreed to take primary responsibility for locating a consultant who could help the team achieve the desired change.

Priority

After completing the first four columns of your Action Plan form, you will need to review and prioritize your desired changes and number each according to its *relative priority* for your program (1 = most important). There might be more than one item to which you want to give a rank of 1. In assigning priorities, the team may want to consider the overall importance of the desired changes to the individual(s) supported in this setting and/or their family members or representatives, the relative importance of the desired changes to the program, and the availability of resources needed (e.g., personnel, funds). Record these relative priority rankings in the fifth column of the Action Plan form. In the previously mentioned example, the overall goal of increasing choices was ranked 1.

When

Once you have agreed on the relative priority for each desired change, you can negotiate the target accomplishment dates for each planned action. Begin with the actions needed to achieve your first-priority goal(s). Write the target completion dates in the last column of your team Action Plan form.

✓✓✓

In the example that we have been following, the team identified two needed actions: scheduling time with a staff member or consultant and increasing the number of choices within each opportunity for choice. Meeting with a staff member or consultant was given a priority of 1 because the team realized that it would not be realistic to try to accomplish this action and increase the number of choices simultaneously. The speech-language pathologist said that she could schedule an initial meeting with the consultant within 3 weeks, so team members set that target date for completing their first action. They planned to take action to increase the number of choices within opportunities for choice 4 weeks after meeting with the consultant.

Because carrying out an Action Plan is an ongoing process, your team needs to maintain regular communication and monitor the achievement of prioritized goals. Your team may also need to make modifications to its Action Plan.

PHOTOCOPYING RELEASE

You may photocopy any part of the *Communication Supports Checklist for Programs Serving Individuals with Severe Disabilities* for distribution for program and staff development and educational purposes. Although photocopying for such purposes is unlimited, no part of the book may be reproduced to generate revenue for any program or individual. Photocopies must be made from an original book.

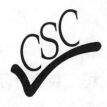

Communication Supports Action Plan

For Programs Serving Individuals with Severe Disabilities

Date Checklist (team consensus rating) completed:

_____

Date Action Plan completed:

_____

Action Plan completed by (list team members and their roles/disciplines):

_____   _____

_____   _____

_____   _____

_____   _____

Section I

Overall Program Support for Communication

A. Philosophy

The following values, attitudes, and beliefs about communication are desirable in all decisions and interactions with individuals with severe disabilities. As a team, we behave in ways that reflect these beliefs:

	Desired Change/Goals	Barriers and Resources	Action Needed	Who	Priority/When
1. Communication is a basic human right.					
2. All individuals should have opportunities to participate fully in their community.					
3. All individuals should have freedom of action and choice.					
4. All individuals communicate in some way; communication may be nonspoken, nonsymbolic, and/or nonintentional.					

A. Philosophy

The following values, attitudes, and beliefs about communication are desirable in all decisions and interactions with individuals with severe disabilities. As a team, we behave in ways that reflect these beliefs:	Desired Change/Goals	Barriers and Resources	Action Needed	Who	Priority/When
5. Appropriate communication goals improve quality of life.					
6. Individuals with severe disabilities and their primary communication partners are involved in communication goal setting and intervention.					
7. Individual and family choices are respected.					
8. Diverse family values and traditions are recognized and respected.					

Communication Supports Checklist • McCarthy et al. • © 1998 Paul H. Brookes Publishing Co., Inc., Baltimore

A. Philosophy

The following values, attitudes, and beliefs about communication are desirable in all decisions and interactions with individuals with severe disabilities. As a team, we behave in ways that reflect these beliefs:

	Desired Change/Goals	Barriers and Resources	Action Needed	Who	Priority/When
9. Team collaboration is essential for effective service.					

B. Protection of Communication Rights

The program ensures the basic communication rights of individuals, regardless of the nature or severity of their disabilities. In the settings being inventoried, communication partners:	Desired Change/Goals	Barriers and Resources	Action Needed	Who	Priority/When
10. Recognize and acknowledge initiations for social interactions.					
11. Recognize and acknowledge requests (for objects, actions, events, people, information, and feedback).					
12. Recognize and acknowledge expressions of feelings and attitudes.					
13. Honor preferences indicated by individuals.					

Communication Supports Checklist • McCarthy et al. • © 1998 Paul H. Brookes Publishing Co., Inc., Baltimore

B. Protection of Communication Rights

(continued)

The program ensures the basic communication rights of individuals, regardless of the nature or severity of their disabilities. In the settings being inventoried, communication partners:	Desired Change/Goals	Barriers and Resources	Action Needed	Who	Priority/When
14. Offer multiple choices in activities throughout the day.					
15. Acknowledge and honor rejections unless the undesired action, event, or object is essential to the individual's protection from harm.					
16. Arrange comprehensive communication assessments and individually appropriate interventions for individuals who might benefit from communication intervention services, regardless of age and severity of disability.					
17. Include peers without disabilities who convey respect and courtesy.					

Communication Supports Checklist • McCarthy et al. • © 1998 Paul H. Brookes Publishing Co., Inc., Baltimore

B.   Protection of Communication Rights

The program ensures the basic communication rights of individuals, regardless of the nature or severity of their disabilities. In the settings being inventoried, communication partners:	Desired Change/Goals	Barriers and Resources	Action Needed	Who	Priority/ When
18. Do not discuss an individual in the third person when that individual is present.					
19. Ensure that individuals have access to assistive technology (AT), augmentative and alternative communication (AAC) devices, and support systems needed for communication at all times.					
20. Ensure that AT and AAC devices are in good working order at all times.					
21. Offer information and explanations when appropriate (e.g., introductions to a classroom or jobsite visitor, explanation about the need to change a planned activity).					

Communication Supports Checklist • McCarthy et al. • © 1998 Paul H. Brookes Publishing Co., Inc., Baltimore

C. Environmental Support for Communication

The environments in which people learn, live, play, and work should promote and support communication. People in each of our program's settings do so by:	Desired Change/Goals	Barriers and Resources	Action Needed	Who	Priority/When
22. Expecting communication (e.g., waiting for an initiation or a response, maintaining visual contact).					
23. Providing interesting and age-appropriate materials, communication partners, and activities.					
24. Following policies and practices that do not prohibit or restrict communication.					
25. Including communication partners who know how to use AAC systems and devices used by individuals (e.g., American Sign Language, graphic symbols, high- and low-technology devices).					

Communication Supports Checklist • McCarthy et al. • © 1998 Paul H. Brookes Publishing Co., Inc., Baltimore

C. Environmental Support for Communication

The environments in which people learn, live, play, and work should promote and support communication. People in each of our program's settings do so by:	Desired Change/Goals	Barriers and Resources	Action Needed	Who	Priority/When
26. Arranging materials so individuals without symbolic communication skills can indicate their interests or requests through the use of gaze, natural gestures, and/or vocal or behavioral signals.					
27. Including peers without disabilities who are available for communication interactions.					
28. Including communication partners who use appropriate language (e.g., primary language) and appropriate communication mode(s) (e.g., oral, signed, graphic, adapted for vision or hearing impairments).					

Communication Supports Checklist • McCarthy et al. • © 1998 Paul H. Brookes Publishing Co., Inc., Baltimore

Section II

Assessment Practices, Goal-Setting Practices, and Program Implementation

A. Assessment Practices

Communication interactions should be observed carefully before program implementation is designed. The degree to which settings are sensitive and responsive to each person's communication needs should also be observed. Goals can be chosen for individuals and the places where they learn, live, play, and work. When assessing an individual's communication abilities and needs, team members:

	Desired Change/Goals	Barriers and Resources	Action Needed	Who	Priority/When
29. Describe the individual's current communication modes (including intentional, nonintentional, symbolic, and nonsymbolic communication).					
30. Include measures of sensory responsivity (i.e., hearing and vision tests) by appropriate professionals.					
31. Include measures of physical status (e.g., positioning, sensorimotor, joint range of motion, motor control) by appropriate professionals.					
32. Identify social functions (e.g., comment, protest, request) of communication behavior across settings.					

Communication Supports Checklist • McCarthy et al. • © 1998 Paul H. Brookes Publishing Co., Inc., Baltimore

A. Assessment Practices

Communication interactions should be observed carefully before program implementation is designed. The degree to which settings are sensitive and responsive to each person's communication needs should also be observed. Goals can be chosen for individuals and the places where they learn, live, play, and work. When assessing an individual's communication abilities and needs, team members:

	Desired Change/Goals	Barriers and Resources	Action Needed	Who	Priority/When
33. Identify the individual's primary communication partners.					
34. Conduct multiple observations over time.					
35. Measure the responsiveness of partners to communication acts.					
36. Measure opportunities for communication across environments (e.g., education, living, leisure, work).					

Communication Supports Checklist • McCarthy et al. • © 1998 Paul H. Brookes Publishing Co., Inc., Baltimore

A. Assessment Practices

Communication interactions should be observed carefully before program implementation is designed. The degree to which settings are sensitive and responsive to each person's communication needs should also be observed. Goals can be chosen for individuals and the places where they learn, live, play, and work. When assessing an individual's communication abilities and needs, team members:

	Desired Change/Goals	Barriers and Resources	Action Needed	Who	Priority/ When
37. Identify the specific communication forms and uses in various modes (e.g., speech, writing, AAC) that are useful across settings.					
38. Measure the spontaneity of communication.					
39. Use a team model that includes the individual, family members, peers, friends, professionals, support personnel, and other significant communication partners.					
40. Specifically ask family members to provide information about perceived communication needs.					

A. Assessment Practices

(continued)

Communication interactions should be observed carefully before program implementation is designed. The degree to which settings are sensitive and responsive to each person's communication needs should also be observed. Goals can be chosen for individuals and the places where they learn, live, play, and work. When assessing an individual's communication abilities and needs, team members:

	Desired Change/Goals	Barriers and Resources	Action Needed	Who	Priority/ When
41. Provide explanations of assessment procedures and results in a way that is meaningful to all team members, including the individual with severe disabilities.					
42. Provide information about communication needs that partners notice during their activities and interactions with individuals.					

Communication Supports Checklist • McCarthy et al. • © 1998 Paul H. Brookes Publishing Co., Inc., Baltimore

Action Plan Section II   CSC   61

B. Goal-Setting Practices

When reaching consensus on appropriate and attainable program implementation goals for an individual, the team:	Desired Change/Goals	Barriers and Resources	Action Needed	Who	Priority/ When
43. Selects and prioritizes goals based on their importance and potential impact on an individual's quality of life.					
44. Uses a team model that includes the individual as well as family members, peers, friends, professionals, support personnel, and other significant communication partners during the planning and implementation of communication interventions.					
45. Considers environmental as well as individual goals.					
46. Takes into account an individual's existing intentional (e.g., pointing to a picture display) and/or nonintentional (e.g., crying) communication abilities.					

Communication Supports Checklist • McCarthy et al. • © 1998 Paul H. Brookes Publishing Co., Inc., Baltimore

B. Goal-Setting Practices

(continued)

When reaching consensus on appropriate and attainable program implementation goals for an individual, the team:	Desired Change/Goals	Barriers and Resources	Action Needed	Who	Priority/When
47. Selects goals consistent with a logical hierarchy of skills and identifies short-term objectives that seem realistically attainable for an individual within a specified time frame (e.g., 6 months, 1 year).					
48. Selects short-term objectives that are consistent with the long-term goals for an individual.					
49. Selects goals that will support an individual's transition to a new environment (e.g., from school to work).					
50. Reviews information from previous teams to ensure continuity of an individual's goals (e.g., person worked on two-choice picture-pointing skills in previous program as a step toward use of a more complex communication board. In new program, team agrees to move on to three-choice picture board).					

Communication Supports Checklist • McCarthy et al. • © 1998 Paul H. Brookes Publishing Co., Inc., Baltimore

C. Program Implementation

Program implementation is based on assessment and selected functional communication goals across settings. Ongoing evaluation is used to measure outcomes and adjust practices accordingly. When implementing intervention programs, the team:

	Desired Change/Goals	Barriers and Resources	Action Needed	Who	Priority/When
51. Targets communication goals primarily in an individual's natural environments during typical interactions, rather than in isolated environments.					
52. Uses pull-out intervention only when necessary for additional practice.					
53. Provides opportunities for initiation, maintenance, and termination of communication/ social interactions.					
54. Provides opportunities to communicate across all environments.					

C. Program Implementation

Program implementation is based on assessment and selected functional communication goals across settings. Ongoing evaluation is used to measure outcomes and adjust practices accordingly. When implementing intervention programs, the team:

	Desired Change/Goals	Barriers and Resources	Action Needed	Who	Priority/When
55. Uses an individual's current communication systems while promoting new skill acquisition.					
56. Uses communication supports and systems that are appropriate to each individual's physical abilities.					
57. Uses communication supports and systems that are appropriate to each individual's sensory abilities.					
58. Uses communication supports and systems that are appropriate to each individual's cognitive abilities.					

C. Program Implementation
(continued)

Program implementation is based on assessment and selected functional communication goals across settings. Ongoing evaluation is used to measure outcomes and adjust practices accordingly. When implementing intervention programs, the team:

	Desired Change/Goals	Barriers and Resources	Action Needed	Who	Priority/When
59. Uses communication supports and systems that are appropriate to an individual's communication needs and environments across settings.					
60. Includes necessary adaptations or modifications to the environment to optimize an individual's use of communication supports and systems (e.g., mounting AAC device on wheelchair).					
61. Provides for the seating and positioning needs of individuals who use communication supports and systems.					
62. Makes assistive devices available to help individuals use supports for communication (e.g., hand/wrist splint, head-controlled pointer, control switches).					

C. Program Implementation

Program implementation is based on assessment and selected functional communication goals across settings. Ongoing evaluation is used to measure outcomes and adjust practices accordingly. When implementing intervention programs, the team:

	Desired Change/Goals	Barriers and Resources	Action Needed	Who	Priority/ When
63. Integrates elements of individual instruction by all team members involved.					
64. Implements plans as designed to accomplish stated goals.					
65. Uses a team model that includes the individual, family members, friends, peers, professionals, support personnel, and other significant communication partners.					
66. Builds on goals and strategies developed in previous programs.					

C. Program Implementation

(continued)

Program implementation is based on assessment and selected functional communication goals across settings. Ongoing evaluation is used to measure outcomes and adjust practices accordingly. When implementing intervention programs, the team:

	Desired Change/Goals	Barriers and Resources	Action Needed	Who	Priority/When
67. Includes and implements plans for continuity and transfer of information regarding communication supports and services before an individual changes program placement.					
68. Includes a specific time schedule for team reassessment of all program elements.					

Section III

Team Competencies

A. Knowledge

CSC

Collectively, the team's knowledge supports and encourages communication. At least one team member has knowledge about:	Desired Change/Goals	Barriers and Resources	Action Needed	Who	Priority/When
69. Human development.					
70. Communication development, including reading and writing.					
71. Individuals with severe disabilities across ages and levels of independence.					
72. Factors that prevent secondary conditions that interfere with communication (e.g., swallowing disorders, poor positioning, challenging behavior).					

Communication Supports Checklist • McCarthy et al. • © 1998 Paul H. Brookes Publishing Co., Inc., Baltimore

A. Knowledge

(continued)

Collectively, the team's knowledge supports and encourages communication. At least one team member has knowledge about:

	Desired Change/Goals	Barriers and Resources	Action Needed	Who	Priority/ When
73. Different means of communication (e.g., body posture, vocalization, gaze, gesture, sign language, electronic and nonelectronic systems).					
74. Different types of communication symbols (e.g., pictures, braille, words, signs, speech).					
75. Amplification and other AT useful to people who have severe disabilities with accompanying sensory limitations.					
76. Medications and their effects on behavior, especially communication.					

Communication Supports Checklist • McCarthy et al. • © 1998 Paul H. Brookes Publishing Co., Inc., Baltimore

A. Knowledge

Collectively, the team's knowledge supports and encourages communication. At least one team member has knowledge about:

	Desired Change/Goals	Barriers and Resources	Action Needed	Who	Priority/When
77. Motor control, muscle tone, and positioning as these affect communication.					
78. Disabilities that may co-occur with communication disorders (e.g., feeding and swallowing problems, seizures, sensory impairments).					
79. Challenging behavior as a potential communication act.					
80. Designing and working with a variety of service delivery models (e.g., classroom-based, pull-out, collaborative).					

A. Knowledge

Collectively, the team's knowledge supports and encourages communication. At least one team member has knowledge about:	Desired Change/Goals	Barriers and Resources	Action Needed	Who	Priority/ When
81. Family dynamics and the impact of severe disability on the family.					
82. The importance of incorporating current research findings into assessment and program implementation.					

Communication Supports Checklist • McCarthy et al. • © 1998 Paul H. Brookes Publishing Co., Inc., Baltimore

B. Skills and Experience

Team members' skills, experiences, and access to resources support and encourage communication. At least one team member has demonstrated the expertise or has the help of resource people who know how to:

	Desired Change/Goals	Barriers and Resources	Action Needed	Who	Priority/When
83. Integrate the domains of cognitive, motor, sensory, and social functioning in communication *assessment* and *goal setting*.					
84. Integrate the domains of cognitive, motor, sensory, and social functioning in communication *implementation*.					
85. Provide ongoing assessment and evaluation using standardized and nonstandardized (formal or informal) procedures.					
86. Plan and implement communication assessments that lead directly to functional communication intervention goals and objectives.					

Communication Supports Checklist • McCarthy et al. • © 1998 Paul H. Brookes Publishing Co., Inc., Baltimore

B. Skills and Experience

(continued)

Team members' skills, experiences, and access to resources support and encourage communication. At least one team member has demonstrated the expertise or has the help of resource people who know how to:	Desired Change/Goals	Barriers and Resources	Action Needed	Who	Priority/When
87. Describe and document functional communication abilities and needs within specific contexts (e.g., educational settings, living environments, recreational environments, vocational environments, the community at large).					
88. Plan, implement, monitor, and modify, as needed, intervention programs that allow individuals to develop functional communication skills in spoken or AAC modes appropriate to educational, living, recreational, and work environments.					
89. Assess emergent and functional literacy skills across all environments.					
90. Teach emergent and functional literacy skills across all environments.					

Communication Supports Checklist • McCarthy et al. • © 1998 Paul H. Brookes Publishing Co., Inc., Baltimore

B. Skills and Experience

Team members' skills, experiences, and access to resources support and encourage communication. At least one team member has demonstrated the expertise or has the help of resource people who know how to:

	Desired Change/Goals	Barriers and Resources	Action Needed	Who	Priority/When
91. Help the individual use the most appropriate (and least intrusive) positioning and mobility aids to maximize functional communication across a variety of environments.					
92. Manage activities of daily living and incorporate functional communication into each of these activities.					
93. Integrate cognition; oral and written communication; and motor, sensory, and social development in defining and implementing communication goals.					
94. Incorporate current research findings into assessment and program implementation.					

B. Skills and Experience

(continued)

Team members' skills, experiences, and access to resources support and encourage communication. At least one team member has demonstrated the expertise or has the help of resource people who know how to:	Desired Change/Goals	Barriers and Resources	Action Needed	Who	Priority/When
95. Promote team participation and self-advocacy on the part of individuals with severe disabilities.					
96. Interact in a culturally sensitive manner.					
97. Understand laws that protect the rights of people with severe disabilities.					

Example #1

A Residential Center

The following Checklist and Action Plan were completed by members of a team working at Sundale Living Center, a residential center for people with developmental disabilities located in a rural part of the southeastern United States. Sundale serves individuals across the age range who have severe multiple disabilities including mental retardation requiring extensive or pervasive support, cerebral palsy, and sensory impairments. The individuals living at Sundale come from diverse socioeconomic and ethnic backgrounds.

The Sundale staff includes specialists from every allied health and habilitation discipline as well as advocates. The center's Checklist and Action Plan were created with input from a qualified developmental disabilities professional (QDDP) who acted as team leader, an advocate, an occupational therapist, a psychologist, a special education teacher, and speech-language pathologists. Team members have had 10–30 years of experience working with individuals who have disabilities.

While completing the forms, the team found room for improvement in three main areas: assessment processes, integration of services across settings, and behavioral interventions. Also, extensive downsizing has caused a shortage of SLPs. Team members noted that completing the Checklist and Action Plan helped involve the SLPs as an integral part of the team.

Example #1   CSC   79

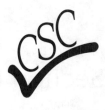

Communication Supports Checklist

For Programs Serving Individuals with Severe Disabilities

Check one: ☐ Individual member rating   ☑ Team consensus rating

Program(s) and/or setting(s) evaluated: Date:

Sundale Living Center: Living Area   _3/16/98_

Checklist completed by (list individual rater or team members and their roles/disciplines):

Lisa Clark, QDDP/team leader	_Kelly Morgan, SLP_
Rowan Johnson, special education teacher	_Denise Esguerra, direct services provider_
Sean Lindo, psychologist	_Beth Chao, advocate_
Lara Singh, SLP	_Anika Jamison, nurse_

Communication Supports Checklist • McCarthy et al. • © 1998 Paul H. Brookes Publishing Co., Inc., Baltimore

Example #1 / Checklist   CSC   81

Section I

Overall Program Support for Communication

Instructions for Rating Items in this Section

When evaluating the program's Overall Program Support for Communication, your team should consider how much program policies, decisions, and practices reflect the values, attitudes, and beliefs listed in Parts A, B, and C of this section. Consider the program's written policies and routine practices as you evaluate these items. A rating of **Consistently True** means that this indicator is true of the attitudes and practices of virtually everyone who interacts with individuals served by the program. A rating of **Sometimes True** should be assigned if you feel that many (but not all) of the staff practices and agency policies are consistent with the attitude or belief identified in an item. A rating of **Rarely True** indicates that a particular attitude or value is rarely or never reflected in the program's routine policies and practices with individuals who have severe disabilities.

A. Philosophy

CSC

The following values, attitudes, and beliefs about communication are desirable in all decisions and interactions with individuals with severe disabilities. As a team, we behave in ways that reflect these beliefs:	Consistently True	Sometimes True	Rarely True	COMMENTS
1. Communication is a basic human right.		✔		We are headed in the right direction, but our behavior does not always reflect this. We take shortcuts for efficiency. Constant staff turnover also prevents transfer of philosophy to new staff.
2. All individuals should have opportunities to participate fully in their community.		✔		Participation is consistent on grounds of facility. It is much more limited in larger community. There are transportation and sometimes access difficulties—our efforts continue in these areas.
3. All individuals should have freedom of action and choice.	✔			Freedom of action and choice has been recognized as a major issue, & currently we are addressing this through person-centered planning.
4. All individuals communicate in some way; communication may be nonspoken, nonsymbolic, and/or nonintentional.	✔			Recognition of this is built into person-centered planning.

Example #1 / Checklist Section I   CSC   83

A. Philosophy

The following values, attitudes, and beliefs about communication are desirable in all decisions and interactions with individuals with severe disabilities. As a team, we behave in ways that reflect these beliefs:	Consistently True	Sometimes True	Rarely True	COMMENTS
5. Appropriate communication goals improve quality of life.		✔		*Since our last self-evaluation, a communication program for every resident has been put in place. Many times the chosen goals feel artificial and do not always contribute to the quality of life of the individual.*
6. Individuals with severe disabilities and their primary communication partners are involved in communication goal setting and intervention.		✔		*This does not always happen across settings with communication partners.*
7. Individual and family choices are respected.	✔			*Always!*
8. Diverse family values and traditions are recognized and respected.		✔		*This sometimes "gets lost in the shuffle" for people who have lived here for a long time. As much as we are aware, we do respect cultural values & traditions.*

Communication Supports Checklist • McCarthy et al. • © 1998 Paul H. Brookes Publishing Co., Inc., Baltimore

A. Philosophy

(continued)

The following values, attitudes, and beliefs about communication are desirable in all decisions and interactions with individuals with severe disabilities. As a team, we behave in ways that reflect these beliefs:	Consistently True	Sometimes True	Rarely True	COMMENTS
9. Team collaboration is essential for effective service.		✓		We believe in collaboration but don't always practice it because of time limitations & logistical factors.

B. Protection of Communication Rights

The program ensures the basic communication rights of individuals, regardless of the nature or severity of their disabilities. In the settings being inventoried, communication partners:	Consistently True	Sometimes True	Rarely True	COMMENTS
10. Recognize and acknowledge initiations for social interactions.		✓		*Recognition of initiations is more likely to happen when the individual is persistent and when there are enough staff members present. Sometimes staffing patterns make it difficult.*
11. Recognize and acknowledge requests (for objects, actions, events, people, information, and feedback).		✓		*Sometimes these requests are weak and fleeting. Sometimes staff members are new & don't recognize the requests, or sometimes the forms used to request things are inappropriate.*
12. Recognize and acknowledge expressions of feelings and attitudes.		✓		*Sometimes staff members don't recognize expressed feelings and attitudes—see #11.*
13. Honor preferences indicated by individuals.		✓		*Most of the time preferences are recognized. Sometimes they are honored to a fault. If a person turns down coleslaw once, it is never offered again!*

Communication Supports Checklist • McCarthy et al. • © 1998 Paul H. Brookes Publishing Co., Inc., Baltimore

B. Protection of Communication Rights

(continued)

The program ensures the basic communication rights of individuals, regardless of the nature or severity of their disabilities. In the settings being inventoried, communication partners:	Consistently True	Sometimes True	Rarely True	COMMENTS
14. Offer multiple choices in activities throughout the day.			✓	*Progress is being made here with current efforts to change day & evening activities. We don't do enough to expose individuals to new things. We need to learn to offer choices in ways that individuals can understand.*
15. Acknowledge and honor rejections unless the undesired action, event, or object is essential to the individual's protection from harm.		✓		*It is hard for staff to handle management of rejections. They are often labeled "noncompliant" and are dealt with as "challenging behavior." Efforts to improve are in progress.*
16. Arrange comprehensive communication assessments and individually appropriate interventions for individuals who might benefit from communication intervention services, regardless of age and severity of disability.		✓		*We have no assessment limitations based on severity of disability or age. However, a shortage of SLPs can and does cause shortcuts in the assessment process.*
17. Include peers without disabilities who convey respect and courtesy.			✓	*In spite of efforts to improve, individuals have the most contact with staff & less contact with peers.*

Communication Supports Checklist • McCarthy et al. • © 1998 Paul H. Brookes Publishing Co., Inc., Baltimore

Example #1 / Checklist Section I   CSC   87

B. Protection of Communication Rights

The program ensures the basic communication rights of individuals, regardless of the nature or severity of their disabilities. In the settings being inventoried, communication partners:	Consistently True	Sometimes True	Rarely True	COMMENTS
18. Do not discuss an individual in the third person when that individual is present.		✓		*This is inconsistent and varies across settings. There is a need for staff training & monitoring so that staff members do not "talk around" individuals.*
19. Ensure that individuals have access to assistive technology (AT), augmentative and alternative communication (AAC) devices, and support systems needed for communication at all times.		✓		*Sometimes AT doesn't work or isn't available. Sometimes staff support could be improved.*
20. Ensure that AT and AAC devices are in good working order at all times.			✓	*This is improving. To improve device functioning, we're working on logistics, staff training/awareness, & communication across settings.*
21. Offer information and explanations when appropriate (e.g., introductions to a classroom or jobsite visitor, explanation about the need to change a planned activity).	✓			*Usually explanations of changes are made, but introductions of different people don't always happen across settings.*

C. Environmental Support for Communication

The environments in which people learn, live, play, and work should promote and support communication. People in each of our program's settings do so by:	Consistently True	Sometimes True	Rarely True	COMMENTS
22. Expecting communication (e.g., waiting for an initiation or a response, maintaining visual contact).	✓			*Much better—staff waits for communication more often than before. The trend is in the right direction, but there is room to improve with people who are not strong communicators.*
23. Providing interesting and age-appropriate materials, communication partners, and activities.	✓			*Efforts are made with materials, but the availability of partners is a concern.*
24. Following policies and practices that do not prohibit or restrict communication.	✓			*During behavioral interventions we need to consider the communication functions of challenging behavior and include communication instruction.*
25. Including communication partners who know how to use AAC systems and devices used by individuals (e.g., American Sign Language, graphic symbols, high- and low-technology devices).	✓			*Turnover creates difficulties with continuity—not all new staff members are familiar with the operation of communication devices and systems used by individuals.*

Communication Supports Checklist • McCarthy et al. • © 1998 Paul H. Brookes Publishing Co., Inc., Baltimore

Example #1 / Checklist Section I   CSC   89

C. Environmental Support for Communication *(continued)*

The environments in which people learn, live, play, and work should promote and support communication. People in each of our program's settings do so by:	Consistently True	Sometimes True	Rarely True	COMMENTS
26. Arranging materials so individuals without symbolic communication skills can indicate their interests or requests through the use of gaze, natural gestures, and/or vocal or behavioral signals.	✓			*Materials are preselected by staff & must be continually arranged and rearranged. Sometimes staff are not available to do so, and sometimes the environments are not conducive to rearranging materials.*
27. Including peers without disabilities who are available for communication interactions.			✓	*Including peers without disabilities is an ongoing concern.*
28. Including communication partners who use appropriate language (e.g., primary language) and appropriate communication mode(s) (e.g., oral, signed, graphic, adapted for vision or hearing impairments).	✓			*There is a need to further explore the use of objects as symbols.*

Communication Supports Checklist • McCarthy et al. • © 1998 Paul H. Brookes Publishing Co., Inc., Baltimore

Section II

Assessment Practices,
Goal-Setting Practices, and Program Implementation

Instructions for Rating Items in this Section

When evaluating the program's Assessment Practices, Goal-Setting Practices, and Program Implementation, your team should consider whether and how much the program's actual practices are consistent with the ideal practices identified in Parts A, B, and C of this section. Consider the program's written procedural policies and routine practices as you consider these items. When rating each item, a rating of **Consistently True** means the statement is consistently true of the practices used by all people involved in communication assessment, goal setting, and program implementation. A rating of **Sometimes True** might indicate some efforts to adopt the practices in the program or that one or two staff members in the program do use the practices. A rating of **Rarely True** indicates that a particular practice is rarely or never reflected in the way that communication needs and abilities are assessed, the way that goals are established, and/or the way that a program is implemented for individuals with severe disabilities served by your program.

Example #1 / Checklist Section II   CSC   91

A. Assessment Practices

Communication interactions should be observed carefully before program implementation is designed. The degree to which settings are sensitive and responsive to each person's communication needs should also be observed. Goals can be chosen for individuals and the places where they learn, live, play, and work. When assessing an individual's communication abilities and needs, team members:

	Consistently True	Sometimes True	Rarely True	COMMENTS
29. Describe the individual's current communication modes (including intentional, nonintentional, symbolic, and non-symbolic communication).	✓			
30. Include measures of sensory responsivity (i.e., hearing and vision tests) by appropriate professionals.	✓			
31. Include measures of physical status (e.g., positioning, sensorimotor, joint range of motion, motor control) by appropriate professionals.	✓			
32. Identify social functions (e.g., comment, protest, request) of communication behavior across settings.		✓		*Up to this point, the focus has been almost totally on requests. We are beginning to address assessment of communication forms and modes, but it is not always done across settings.*

Communication Supports Checklist • McCarthy et al. • © 1998 Paul H. Brookes Publishing Co., Inc., Baltimore

A. Assessment Practices

Communication interactions should be observed carefully before program implementation is designed. The degree to which settings are sensitive and responsive to each person's communication needs should also be observed. Goals can be chosen for individuals and the places where they learn, live, play, and work. When assessing an individual's communication abilities and needs, team members:	Consistently True	Sometimes True	Rarely True	COMMENTS
33. Identify the individual's primary communication partners.	✓			
34. Conduct multiple observations over time.		✓		*Teachers & direct services staff observe daily. An SLP is not always an integral part of the team and should conduct more observation over time and across settings.*
35. Measure the responsiveness of partners to communication acts.		✓		*Partner responsiveness is monitored with supervisory and quality improvement tools but usually is not looked at as part of the assessment process.*
36. Measure opportunities for communication across environments (e.g., education, leisure, living, work).		✓		*Efforts to generalize assessments to more than one setting are made but are still not consistent or comprehensive. Challenges include staffing patterns, time constraints, and thinking "in the box."*

Communication Supports Checklist • McCarthy et al. • © 1998 Paul H. Brookes Publishing Co., Inc., Baltimore

Example #1 / Checklist Section II   CSC   93

A.   Assessment Practices

Communication interactions should be observed carefully before program implementation is designed. The degree to which settings are sensitive and responsive to each person's communication needs should also be observed. Goals can be chosen for individuals and the places where they learn, live, play, and work. When assessing an individual's communication abilities and needs, team members:

	Consistently True	Sometimes True	Rarely True	COMMENTS
37. Identify the specific communication forms and uses in various modes (e.g., speech, writing, AAC) that are useful across settings.		✔		*We tend to try to teach more symbols rather than expand across settings.*
38. Measure the spontaneity of communication.		✔		*We have talked about this in some detail—we have differing perceptions of what "spontaneous" means.*
39. Use a team model that includes the individual, family members, peers, friends, professionals, support personnel, and other significant communication partners.	✔			
40. Specifically ask family members to provide information about perceived communication needs.	✔			

A. Assessment Practices

Communication interactions should be observed carefully before program implementation is designed. The degree to which settings are sensitive and responsive to each person's communication needs should also be observed. Goals can be chosen for individuals and the places where they learn, live, play, and work. When assessing an individual's communication abilities and needs, team members:

	Consistently True	Sometimes True	Rarely True	COMMENTS
41. Provide explanations of assessment procedures and results in ways that are meaningful to all team members, including the individual with severe disabilities.		✓		*Explanations of assessment procedures are sometimes given but are not as meaningful as they might be. Demonstrations would be more effective than words for direct services staff.*
42. Provide information about communication needs that partners notice during their activities and interactions with individuals.		✓		*Communication needs are frequently observed in isolated, specific settings.*

Example #1 / Checklist Section II   CSC   95

B.   Goal-Setting Practices

CSC ✓

When reaching consensus on appropriate and attainable program implementation goals for an individual, the team:	Consistently True	Sometimes True	Rarely True	COMMENTS
43. Selects and prioritizes goals based on their importance and potential impact on an individual's quality of life.	✓			*Although interventions are sometimes isolated and situation-specific, we <u>do</u> choose things to target that are important to the individual.*
44. Uses a team model that includes the individual as well as family members, peers, friends, professionals, support personnel, and other significant communication partners during the planning and implementation of communication interventions.		✓		*Communication is almost always discussed at team meetings, but sometimes unilateral decisions are made to change interventions without involving all team members.*
45. Considers environmental as well as individual goals.		✓		*Environmental and individual goals are considered in some environments but not in others. Changes now in progress should help improve this.*
46. Takes into account an individual's existing intentional (e.g., pointing to a picture display) and/or nonintentional (e.g., crying) communication abilities.	✓			

Communication Supports Checklist • McCarthy et al. • © 1998 Paul H. Brookes Publishing Co., Inc., Baltimore

B. Goal-Setting Practices

(continued)

When reaching consensus on appropriate and attainable program implementation goals for an individual, the team:	Consistently True	Sometimes True	Rarely True	COMMENTS
47. Selects goals consistent with a logical hierarchy of skills and identifies short-term objectives that seem realistically attainable for an individual within a specified time frame (e.g., 6 months, 1 year).	✓			
48. Selects short-term objectives that are consistent with the long-term goals for an individual.	✓			
49. Selects goals that will support an individual's transition to a new environment (e.g., from school to work).		✓		*Often we don't know very much in advance what the next environment will be, and we either don't have or don't take the time to study and plan before transitions.*
50. Reviews information from previous teams to ensure continuity of an individual's goals (e.g., person worked on two-choice picture-pointing skills in previous program as a step toward use of a more complex communication board. In new program, team agrees to move on to three-choice picture board).	✓			

Communication Supports Checklist • McCarthy et al. • © 1998 Paul H. Brookes Publishing Co., Inc., Baltimore

Example #1 / Checklist Section II   CSC   97

C. Program Implementation

Program implementation is based on assessment and selected functional communication goals across settings. Ongoing evaluation is used to measure outcomes and adjust practices accordingly. When implementing intervention programs, the team:

	Consistently True	Sometimes True	Rarely True	COMMENTS
51. Targets communication goals primarily in an individual's natural environments during typical interactions, rather than in isolated environments.	✔			
52. Uses pull-out intervention only when necessary for additional practice.	✔			
53. Provides opportunities for initiation, maintenance, and termination of communication/social interactions.		✔		*Our focus has been on requests, which create respondent behavior and only one kind of communication function.*
54. Provides opportunities to communicate across all environments.			✔	*We are still seeing limited opportunities to provide communication across settings.*

Communication Supports Checklist • McCarthy et al. • © 1998 Paul H. Brookes Publishing Co., Inc., Baltimore

C.   Program Implementation

Program implementation is based on assessment and selected functional communication goals across settings. Ongoing evaluation is used to measure outcomes and adjust practices accordingly. When implementing intervention programs, the team:	Consistently True	Sometimes True	Rarely True	COMMENTS
55. Uses an individual's current communication systems while promoting new skill acquisition.	✓			
56. Uses communication supports and systems that are appropriate to each individual's physical abilities.	✓			
57. Uses communication supports and systems that are appropriate to each individual's sensory abilities.	✓			
58. Uses communication supports and systems that are appropriate to each individual's cognitive abilities.		✓		*Sometimes instructions/explanations are too lengthy. We don't use short phrases and key words enough. Symbol set is sometimes not optimal.*

C. Program Implementation

(continued)

Program implementation is based on assessment and selected functional communication goals across settings. Ongoing evaluation is used to measure outcomes and adjust practices accordingly. When implementing intervention programs, the team:	Consistently True	Sometimes True	Rarely True	COMMENTS
59. Uses communication supports and systems that are appropriate to each individual's communication needs and environments across settings.	✓			*Often systems and supports are in place in formal, structured settings but aren't in use in the living area.*
60. Includes necessary adaptations or modifications to the environment to optimize an individual's use of communication supports and systems (e.g., mounting AAC device on wheelchair).	✓			*Again, adaptations are made in formal settings but not in the living area.*
61. Provides for the seating and positioning needs of individuals who use communication supports and systems.				*N/A—All individuals are ambulatory and do not need special positioning devices.*
62. Makes assistive devices available to help individuals use supports for communication (e.g., hand/wrist splint, head-controlled pointer, control switches).				*N/A—See #61.*

C. Program Implementation

Program implementation is based on assessment and selected functional communication goals across settings. Ongoing evaluation is used to measure outcomes and adjust practices accordingly. When implementing intervention programs, the team:

	Consistently True	Sometimes True	Rarely True	COMMENTS
63. Integrates elements of individual instruction by all team members involved.	✓			
64. Implements plans as designed to accomplish stated goals.	✓			
65. Uses a team model that includes the individual, family members, friends, peers, professionals, support personnel, and other significant communication partners.		✓		*Often an audiologist isn't present. Ophthalmologist input comes from nursing staff. SLP involvement could be improved—right now we have a shortage of SLPs.*
66. Builds on goals and strategies developed in previous programs.	✓			

C.   Program Implementation

Program implementation is based on assessment and se-lected functional communication goals across settings. Ongoing evaluation is used to measure outcomes and ad-just practices accordingly. When implementing interven-tion programs, the team:

	Consistently True	Sometimes True	Rarely True	COMMENTS
67. Includes and implements plans for continuity and transfer of information regarding communication supports and services before an individual changes program placement.		✔		*We don't always know in advance when someone is moving internally between different living areas. Sometimes information on admissions is not readily available.*
68. Includes a specific time schedule for team reassessment of all program elements.	✔			

Communication Supports Checklist • McCarthy et al. • © 1998 Paul H. Brookes Publishing Co., Inc., Baltimore

Section III

Team Competencies

Instructions for Rating Items in this Section

Rate the knowledge and skills that team members contribute as combined resources. Specific types of knowledge and skills are identified in Parts A and B of this section. Consider the specific training, experiences, and expertise of each team member, including family members, as you consider these items. When rating these items, a rating of **Consistently True** means that one or more team members has outstanding knowledge, skills, and/or experience relevant to that particular item. A rating of **Sometimes True** should be assigned if you believe that one or two (but not all) team members demonstrate this knowledge or skill. A rating of **Sometimes True** should also be assigned if you have the occasional help of a resource person (not a regular member of the team), but the team agrees that it would be desirable for additional team members to share this knowledge or skill or that the levels of expertise could be improved. A rating of **Rarely True** indicates that a particular knowledge or skill is clearly not demonstrated by any single member of the team.

Example #1 / Checklist Section III   CSC   103

A. Knowledge

Collectively, the team's knowledge supports and encourages communication. At least one team member has knowledge about:	Consistently True	Sometimes True	Rarely True	COMMENTS
69. Human development.	✔			
70. Communication development, including reading and writing.	✔			
71. Individuals with severe disabilities across ages and levels of independence.	✔			*We have residents across the age range, so all team members have this expertise.*
72. Factors that prevent secondary conditions that interfere with communication (e.g., swallowing disorders, poor positioning, challenging behavior).	✔			

A. Knowledge

(continued)

Collectively, the team's knowledge supports and encourages communication. At least one team member has knowledge about:	Consistently True	Sometimes True	Rarely True	COMMENTS
73. Different means of communication (e.g., body posture, vocalization, gaze, gesture, sign language, electronic and nonelectronic systems).	✓			
74. Different types of communication symbols (e.g., pictures, braille, words, signs, speech).	✓			
75. Amplification and other AT useful to people who have severe disabilities with accompanying sensory limitations.	✓			
76. Medications and their effects on behavior, especially communication.		✓		*We have information and expertise on the effects of medication on behavior but not specifically relating to communication.*

Communication Supports Checklist • McCarthy et al. • © 1998 Paul H. Brookes Publishing Co., Inc., Baltimore

Example #1 / Checklist Section III   CSC   105

A. Knowledge

(continued)

Collectively, the team's knowledge supports and encourages communication. At least one team member has knowledge about:	Consistently True	Sometimes True	Rarely True	COMMENTS
77. Motor control, muscle tone, and positioning as these affect communication.	✓			
78. Disabilities that may co-occur with communication disorders (e.g., feeding and swallowing problems, seizures, sensory impairments).		✓		*Information related to vision problems is not readily available.*
79. Challenging behavior as a potential communication act.			✓	*There is not much input related to communication in behavior programs. We are aware of the relationship between communication and challenging behavior but don't always act on it.*
80. Designing and working with a variety of service delivery models (e.g., classroom-based, pull-out, collaborative).	✓			

Communication Supports Checklist • McCarthy et al. • © 1998 Paul H. Brookes Publishing Co., Inc., Baltimore

A. Knowledge

Collectively, the team's knowledge supports and encourages communication. At least one team member has knowledge about:	Consistently True	Sometimes True	Rarely True	COMMENTS
81. Family dynamics and the impact of severe disability on the family.	✓			*Team members have a knowledge of family dynamics, but we could apply this knowledge more often.*
82. The importance of incorporating current research findings into assessment and program implementation.	✓			*There is no consistent mechanism for sharing research from the literature. Individual team members keep up as best they can.*

Communication Supports Checklist • McCarthy et al. • © 1998 Paul H. Brookes Publishing Co., Inc., Baltimore

Example #1 / Checklist Section III   CSC   107

B.   Skills and Experience

Team members' skills, experiences, and access to resources support and encourage communication. At least one team member has demonstrated the expertise or has the help of resource people who know how to:

	Consistently True	Sometimes True	Rarely True	COMMENTS
83. Integrate the domains of cognitive, motor, sensory, and social functioning in communication *assessment* and *goal setting*.	✔			*Social functioning has not been a focus of assessment.*
84. Integrate the domains of cognitive, motor, sensory, and social functioning in communication *implementation*.	✔			*As with #83, social functioning hasn't been a focus in implementation.*
85. Provide ongoing assessment and evaluation using standardized and nonstandardized (formal or informal) procedures.	✔			*There could be more continual ongoing assessment from SLPs.*
86. Plan and implement communication assessments that lead directly to functional communication intervention goals and objectives.	✔			*Interventions don't always follow directly from assessment results.*

B.   Skills and Experience

(continued)

Team members' skills, experiences, and access to resources support and encourage communication. At least one team member has demonstrated the expertise or has the help of resource people who know how to:	Consistently True	Sometimes True	Rarely True	COMMENTS
87. Describe and document functional communication abilities and needs within specific contexts (e.g., educational settings, living environments, recreational environments, vocational environments, the community at large).	✓			*Team members have the expertise, but it is not always put to use.*
88. Plan, implement, monitor, and modify, as needed, intervention programs that allow individuals to develop functional communication skills in spoken or AAC modes appropriate to educational, living, recreational, and work environments.	✓			*Integration of AAC use across settings should be improved.*
89. Assess emergent and functional literacy skills across all environments.	✓			*When the need for literacy assessment is apparent, it is addressed.*
90. Teach emergent and functional literacy skills across all environments.	✓			*Literacy skills are taught as needed.*

Example #1 / Checklist Section III   CSC   109

B. Skills and Experience

(continued)

Team members' skills, experiences, and access to resources support and encourage communication. At least one team member has demonstrated the expertise or has the help of resource people who know how to:	Consistently True	Sometimes True	Rarely True	COMMENTS
91. Help the individual use the most appropriate (and least intrusive) positioning and mobility aids to maximize functional communication across a variety of environments.				*N/A—Individuals don't require special positioning.*
92. Manage activities of daily living and incorporate functional communication into each of these activities.		✓		*We recognize the need to incorporate communication in daily activities, but this area needs improvement.*
93. Integrate cognition; oral and written communication; and motor, sensory, and social development in defining and implementing communication goals.		✓		*As with #92, we recognize the need to consider these aspects of goal setting and implementation, but this area needs improvement.*
94. Incorporate current research findings into assessment and program implementation.		✓		*We have no forum for sharing research, so incorporation of research in assessment & procedures occurs when individual staff members take the initiative.*

B. Skills and Experience

Team members' skills, experiences, and access to resources support and encourage communication. At least one team member has demonstrated the expertise or has the help of resource people who know how to:

	Consistently True	Sometimes True	Rarely True	COMMENTS
95. Promote team participation and self-advocacy on the part of individuals with severe disabilities.	✓			
96. Interact in a culturally sensitive manner. ◄	✓			Team members reported that, as far as they are aware, they interact in ways that respect families' values and traditions (see #8).
97. Understand laws that protect the rights of people with severe disabilities.	✓			

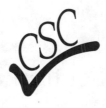

Communication Supports Action Plan

For Programs Serving Individuals with Severe Disabilities

Date Checklist (team consensus rating) completed:

_3/16/98_

Date Action Plan completed:

_3/23/98_

> These five team members provided written input for the Action Plan.

Action Plan completed by (list team members and their roles/disciplines):

Lisa Clark, QDDP/team leader

Beth Chao, advocate

Lara Singh, SLP

Kelly Morgan, SLP

Sean Lindo, psychologist

Rowan Johnson, special education teacher

Denise Esguerra, direct services provider

Sasha Peterson, occupational therapist assistant

Anika Jamison, nurse

Example #1 / Action Plan   CSC   113

Section I

Overall Program Support for Communication

A. Philosophy

The following values, attitudes, and beliefs about communication are desirable in all decisions and interactions with individuals with severe disabilities. As a team, we behave in ways that reflect these beliefs:

	Desired Change/Goals	Barriers and Resources	Action Needed	Who	Priority/When
1. Communication is a basic human right.					
2. All individuals should have opportunities to participate fully in their community.					
3. All individuals should have freedom of action and choice.					
4. All individuals communicate in some way; communication may be nonspoken, nonsymbolic, and/or nonintentional.					

> Freedom of action and choice are being addressed through person-centered planning, a process that has been in place for a short time. Team members reported that staff are still adapting to the new process.

Communication Supports Checklist • McCarthy et al. • © 1998 Paul H. Brookes Publishing Co., Inc., Baltimore

Example #1 / Action Plan Section I   CSC   115

A. Philosophy

(continued)

The following values, attitudes, and beliefs about communication are desirable in all decisions and interactions with individuals with severe disabilities. As a team, we behave in ways that reflect these beliefs:

	Desired Change/Goals	Barriers and Resources	Action Needed	Who	Priority/When
5. Appropriate communication goals improve quality of life.	Tie communication goals directly to assessment results and functional activities.	Many communication instruction objectives for residents involve requesting food. Access to favorite foods is motivating, but the instruction may not improve quality of life.	Continue reorganization of the day program.	Communication Services Director	1 Ongoing
6. Individuals with severe disabilities and their primary communication partners are involved in communication goal setting and intervention.					
7. Individual and family choices are respected.					
8. Diverse family values and traditions are recognized and respected.					

A. Philosophy

The following values, attitudes, and beliefs about communication are desirable in all decisions and interactions with individuals with severe disabilities. As a team, we behave in ways that reflect these beliefs:

	Desired Change/Goals	Barriers and Resources	Action Needed	Who	Priority/When
9. Team collaboration is essential for effective service.	More cross-discipline/cross-setting participation in assessment and goal setting	Time and logistical barriers. We believe it, but it doesn't always translate into practice.	SLPs to increase input to person-centered planning and facilitate integration through contact with staff during direct services provision (at targeted times across day)	SLPs	1 — Early this summer

B. Protection of Communication Rights

The program ensures the basic communication rights of individuals, regardless of the nature or severity of their disabilities. In the settings being inventoried, communication partners:

	Desired Change/Goals	Barriers and Resources	Action Needed	Who	Priority/When
10. Recognize and acknowledge initiations for social interactions.					
11. Recognize and acknowledge requests (for objects, actions, events, people, information, and feedback).					
12. Recognize and acknowledge expressions of feelings and attitudes.					
13. Honor preferences indicated by individuals.		This issue is being addressed through current efforts to teach staff how to handle rejections, including some forms of challenging behavior (see #15 in the Checklist).			

Communication Supports Checklist • McCarthy et al. • © 1998 Paul H. Brookes Publishing Co., Inc., Baltimore

B. Protection of Communication Rights

(continued)

The program ensures the basic communication rights of individuals, regardless of the nature or severity of their disabilities. In the settings being inventoried, communication partners:	Desired Change/Goals	Barriers and Resources	Action Needed	Who	Priority/When
14. Offer multiple choices in activities throughout the day.	Offer choices in ways that individual can understand. Honor right to refuse all options given.	Lack of knowledge, staff shortages	Provide additional staff training; provide support with ancillary staff.	QDDP, SLPs, ancillary staff	1 — Begin staff training by early summer.
15. Acknowledge and honor rejections unless the undesired action, event, or object is essential to the individual's protection from harm.					
16. Arrange comprehensive communication assessments and individually appropriate interventions for individuals who might benefit from communication intervention services, regardless of age and severity of disability.	Increase the comprehensive nature of assessment.	Severe shortage of SLPs has caused shortcuts in the assessment process.	SLPs to focus on direct gathering of information for input to person-centered plans rather than relying heavily on others' reports	SLPs and QDDP	1 — Start now. It will take a year to cycle through all plans.
17. Include peers without disabilities who convey respect and courtesy.					

B. Protection of Communication Rights

The program ensures the basic communication rights of individuals, regardless of the nature or severity of their disabilities. In the settings being inventoried, communication partners:	Desired Change/Goals	Barriers and Resources	Action Needed	Who	Priority/ When
18. Do not discuss an individual in the third person when that individual is present.					
19. Ensure that individuals have access to assistive technology (AT), augmentative and alternative communication (AAC) devices, and support systems needed for communication at all times.	*Improve access to AT and support systems.*	*Shortage of knowledgeable, experienced staff*	*1) Train key staff so they can support SLPs. 2) Create a compensatory education program at community college, focusing on AT integration across settings.*	*1) SLPs, AT resource specialist 2) Communication Services Director, SLPs, Education Director*	*1*	*Begin by early June.*
20. Ensure that AT and AAC devices are in good working order at all times.	*Improve identification & reporting of equipment breakdowns and response times for repairs.*	*Staff shortages, failure to report breakdowns*	*Review system for reporting equipment breakdowns, communicate procedure to QDDP and direct care supervisors, and identify additional resources.*	*AAC specialist, AAC equipment technician, & AT resource specialist*	*1*	*Begin by late spring.*
21. Offer information and explanations when appropriate (e.g., introductions to a classroom or jobsite visitor, explanation about the need to change a planned activity).					

C. Environmental Support for Communication

The environments in which people learn, live, play, and work should promote and support communication. People in each of our program's settings do so by:

	Desired Change/Goals	Barriers and Resources	Action Needed	Who	Priority/When
22. Expecting communication (e.g., waiting for an initiation or a response, maintaining visual contact).					
23. Providing interesting and age-appropriate materials, communication partners, and activities.					
24. Following policies and practices that do not prohibit or restrict communication.					
25. Including communication partners who know how to use AAC systems and devices used by individuals (e.g., American Sign Language, graphic symbols, high- and low-technology devices).					

> Obtaining materials is usually not difficult, but providing communication partners has been an ongoing concern. The team, however, decided to address this issue at another time.

C. Environmental Support for Communication *(continued)*

The environments in which people learn, live, play, and work should promote and support communication. People in each of our program's settings do so by:	Desired Change/Goals	Barriers and Resources	Action Needed	Who	Priority/ When
26. Arranging materials so individuals without symbolic communication skills can indicate their interests or requests through the use of gaze, natural gestures, and/or vocal or behavioral signals.					
27. Including peers without disabilities who are available for communication interactions.					
28. Including communication partners who use appropriate language (e.g., primary language) and appropriate communication mode(s) (e.g., oral, signed, graphic, adapted for vision or hearing impairments).					

Including peers has been an ongoing concern, but team members did not identify this as a priority to be addressed in their Action Plan at this time.

Communication Supports Checklist • McCarthy et al. • © 1998 Paul H. Brookes Publishing Co., Inc., Baltimore

Section II

Assessment Practices, Goal-Setting Practices, and Program Implementation

Example #1 / Action Plan Section II   CSC   123

A. Assessment Practices

Communication interactions should be observed carefully before program implementation is designed. The degree to which settings are sensitive and responsive to each person's communication needs should also be observed. Goals can be chosen for individuals and the places where they learn, live, play, and work. When assessing an individual's communication abilities and needs, team members:

	Desired Change/Goals	Barriers and Resources	Action Needed	Who	Priority/When
29. Describe the individual's current communication modes (including intentional, nonintentional, symbolic, and nonsymbolic communication).					
30. Include measures of sensory responsivity (i.e., hearing and vision tests) by appropriate professionals.					
31. Include measures of physical status (e.g., positioning, sensorimotor, joint range of motion, motor control) by appropriate professionals.					
32. Identify social functions (e.g., comment, protest, request) of communication behavior across settings.					

The team will begin to address challenging behavior as potential communication during assessments and interventions (see #79).

A. Assessment Practices

Communication interactions should be observed carefully before program implementation is designed. The degree to which settings are sensitive and responsive to each person's communication needs should also be observed. Goals can be chosen for individuals and the places where they learn, live, play, and work. When assessing an individual's communication abilities and needs, team members:

	Desired Change/Goals	Barriers and Resources	Action Needed	Who	Priority/When
33. Identify the individual's primary communication partners.					
34. Conduct multiple observations over time.	Increase SLPs' direct observation of communication behaviors across settings.	Lack of staff	Shift focus of SLPs from creation of paper for individuals' files to more comprehensive assessment for input to person-centered planning.	SLPs and QDDP	1 Start now.
35. Measure the responsiveness of partners to communication acts.	See #34.				
36. Measure opportunities for communication across environments (e.g., education, living, leisure, work).	See #34.				

A. Assessment Practices

Communication interactions should be observed carefully before program implementation is designed. The degree to which settings are sensitive and responsive to each person's communication needs should also be observed. Goals can be chosen for individuals and the places where they learn, live, play, and work. When assessing an individual's communication abilities and needs, team members:

	Desired Change/Goals	Barriers and Resources	Action Needed	Who	Priority/When
37. Identify the specific communication forms and uses in various modes (e.g., speech, writing, AAC) that are useful across settings.	*See #34.*				
38. Measure the spontaneity of communication.					
39. Use a team model that includes the individual, family members, peers, friends, professionals, support personnel, and other significant communication partners.					
40. Specifically ask family members to provide information about perceived communication needs.					

A. Assessment Practices (continued)

Communication interactions should be observed carefully before program implementation is designed. The degree to which settings are sensitive and responsive to each person's communication needs should also be observed. Goals can be chosen for individuals and the places where they learn, live, play, and work. When assessing an individual's communication abilities and needs, team members:

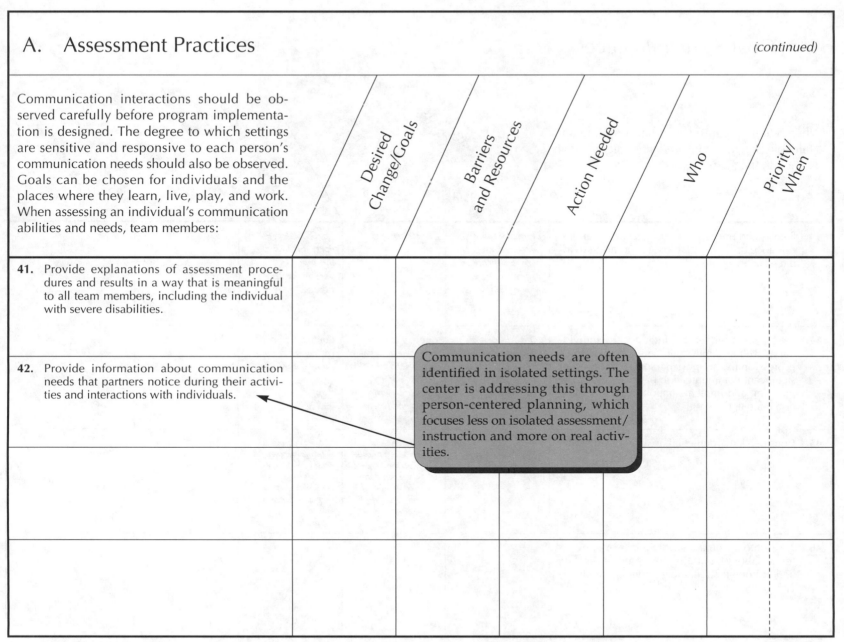

	Desired Change/Goals	Barriers and Resources	Action Needed	Who	Priority/When
41. Provide explanations of assessment procedures and results in a way that is meaningful to all team members, including the individual with severe disabilities.					
42. Provide information about communication needs that partners notice during their activities and interactions with individuals.					

Communication needs are often identified in isolated settings. The center is addressing this through person-centered planning, which focuses less on isolated assessment/instruction and more on real activities.

Example #1 / Action Plan Section II   CSC   127

B. Goal-Setting Practices

When reaching consensus on appropriate and attainable program implementation goals for an individual, the team:	Desired Change/Goals	Barriers and Resources	Action Needed	Who	Priority/When
43. Selects and prioritizes goals based on their importance and potential impact on an individual's quality of life.	Improve input to person-centered planning process regarding communication skills.	Shortage of SLPs	Focus SLP efforts on improving input to person-centered process—see #9.	SLPs	/ Start now.
44. Uses a team model that includes the individual as well as family members, peers, friends, professionals, support personnel, and other significant communication partners during the planning and implementation of communication interventions.	More involvement of peers without disabilities	Lack of contact with peers without disabilities & people not connected by employment to the center	Continue efforts to increase community contacts.	QDDP and team	/ Ongoing
45. Considers environmental as well as individual goals.	Increase attention to environmental goals.	1) A tradition of focusing on skill acquisition at the expense of skill actualization 2) A computer system not designed to track environmental interventions	1) Continue implementing person-centered planning. 2) Implement new computer system that can document environmental supports.	QDDP & team responsible for both	/ Ongoing
46. Takes into account an individual's existing intentional (e.g., pointing to a picture display) and/or nonintentional (e.g., crying) communication abilities.					

B. Goal-Setting Practices *(continued)*

When reaching consensus on appropriate and attainable program implementation goals for an individual, the team:	Desired Change/Goals	Barriers and Resources	Action Needed	Who	Priority/When
47. Selects goals consistent with a logical hierarchy of skills and identifies short-term objectives that seem realistically attainable for an individual within a specified time frame (e.g., 6 months, 1 year).					
48. Selects short-term objectives that are consistent with the long-term goals for an individual.					
49. Selects goals that will support an individual's transition to a new environment (e.g., from school to work).					
50. Reviews information from previous teams to ensure continuity of an individual's goals (e.g., person worked on two-choice picture-pointing skills in previous program as a step toward use of a more complex communication board. In new program, team agrees to move on to three-choice picture board).					

Sometimes the team is not able to plan for transitions because they do not know when an individual is moving between different living areas in the center. The proposed computer system (see #45) should help the team obtain this information further in advance.

Example #1 / Action Plan Section II   CSC   129

C. Program Implementation

Program implementation is based on assessment and selected functional communication goals across settings. Ongoing evaluation is used to measure outcomes and adjust practices accordingly. When implementing intervention programs, the team:

	Desired Change/Goals	Barriers and Resources	Action Needed	Who	Priority/ When
51. Targets communication goals primarily in an individual's natural environments during typical interactions, rather than in isolated environments.					
52. Uses pull-out intervention only when necessary for additional practice.					
53. Provides opportunities for initiation, maintenance, and termination of communication/ social interactions.					
54. Provides opportunities to communicate across all environments.	*Increase opportunities for communication in living area activities.*	*Lack of staff knowledge & lack of well-planned, well-executed activities in living areas*	*Target specific locations and times of the day that are problematic, & focus SLP and teacher efforts on improving those activities.*	*Communication Services Director, SLPs, Education Director, teachers*	*1* *Ongoing*

Communication Supports Checklist • McCarthy et al. • © 1998 Paul H. Brookes Publishing Co., Inc., Baltimore

C.   Program Implementation

Program implementation is based on assessment and selected functional communication goals across settings. Ongoing evaluation is used to measure outcomes and adjust practices accordingly. When implementing intervention programs, the team:

	Desired Change/Goals	Barriers and Resources	Action Needed	Who	Priority/When
55. Uses an individual's current communication systems while promoting new skill acquisition.					
56. Uses communication supports and systems that are appropriate to each individual's physical abilities.					
57. Uses communication supports and systems that are appropriate to each individual's sensory abilities.					
58. Uses communication supports and systems that are appropriate to each individual's cognitive abilities.	*Increase staff understanding of communication development.*	*1) Lack of knowledge about communication development 2) Little sharing of assessment results and their implications with other staff*	*1) Staff training 2) Improve input to person-centered planning.*	*SLPs*	*1* → *1) Develop curriculum by June. 2) Start now.*

C. Program Implementation

Program implementation is based on assessment and selected functional communication goals across settings. Ongoing evaluation is used to measure outcomes and adjust practices accordingly. When implementing intervention programs, the team:

	Desired Change/Goals	Barriers and Resources	Action Needed	Who	Priority/When
59. Uses communication supports and systems that are appropriate to an individual's communication needs and environments across settings.	"Across settings" is where the difficulty lies.	Staff knowledge & shortages	1) Provide additional training. 2) Provide ancillary staff and compensatory education—see #19.	QDDP, SLPs, ancillary staff	*1* — Start staff training this summer.
60. Includes necessary adaptations or modifications to the environment to optimize an individual's use of communication supports and systems (e.g., mounting AAC device on wheelchair).					
61. Provides for the seating and positioning needs of individuals who use communication supports and systems.					
62. Makes assistive devices available to help individuals use supports for communication (e.g., hand/wrist splint, head-controlled pointer, control switches).					

C. Program Implementation

Program implementation is based on assessment and selected functional communication goals across settings. Ongoing evaluation is used to measure outcomes and adjust practices accordingly. When implementing intervention programs, the team:

	Desired Change/Goals	Barriers and Resources	Action Needed	Who	Priority/ When
63. Integrates elements of individual instruction by all team members involved.					
64. Implements plans as designed to accomplish stated goals.					
65. Uses a team model that includes the individual, family members, friends, peers, professionals, support personnel, and other significant communication partners.					
66. Builds on goals and strategies developed in previous programs.					

> Team members said that SLPs could be more involved in team efforts and recognized that recent staff cutbacks have contributed to demands on the SLPs' time. The team plans for SLPs to play a more active role in person-centered planning (see #9).

Communication Supports Checklist • McCarthy et al. • © 1998 Paul H. Brookes Publishing Co., Inc., Baltimore

Example #1 / Action Plan Section II   CSC   133

C. Program Implementation

Program implementation is based on assessment and selected functional communication goals across settings. Ongoing evaluation is used to measure outcomes and adjust practices accordingly. When implementing intervention programs, the team:

	Desired Change/Goals	Barriers and Resources	Action Needed	Who	Priority/When
67. Includes and implements plans for continuity and transfer of information regarding communication supports and services before an individual changes program placement.			As noted in #49, the proposed computer system could help team members find out in advance when individuals will be moving between living areas.		
68. Includes a specific time schedule for team reassessment of all program elements.					

Communication Supports Checklist • McCarthy et al. • © 1998 Paul H. Brookes Publishing Co., Inc., Baltimore

Section III

Team Competencies

Example #1 / Action Plan Section III   CSC   135

A. Knowledge

Collectively, the team's knowledge supports and encourages communication. At least one team member has knowledge about:	Desired Change/Goals	Barriers and Resources	Action Needed	Who	Priority/When
69. Human development.					
70. Communication development, including reading and writing.			One of the team's Action Plan goals is to increase staff members' understanding of communication development so that they can provide communication supports appropriate to each individual's cognitive abilities (see #58).		
71. Individuals with severe disabilities across ages and levels of independence.					
72. Factors that prevent secondary conditions that interfere with communication (e.g., swallowing disorders, poor positioning, challenging behavior).					

A. Knowledge

(continued)

Collectively, the team's knowledge supports and encourages communication. At least one team member has knowledge about:	Desired Change/Goals	Barriers and Resources	Action Needed	Who	Priority/When
73. Different means of communication (e.g., body posture, vocalization, gaze, gesture, sign language, electronic and nonelectronic systems).					
74. Different types of communication symbols (e.g., pictures, braille, words, signs, speech).					
75. Amplification and other AT useful to people who have severe disabilities with accompanying sensory limitations.					
76. Medications and their effects on behavior, especially communication.	Increase team knowledge about effects of medication on behavior & communication.	Lack of knowledge	Contact director of medical services about increasing knowledge in this area..	Communication Services Director	1 — Start now.

Example #1 / Action Plan Section III   CSC   137

A. Knowledge

Collectively, the team's knowledge supports and encourages communication. At least one team member has knowledge about:

	Desired Change/Goals	Barriers and Resources	Action Needed	Who	Priority/When
77. Motor control, muscle tone, and positioning as these affect communication.					
78. Disabilities that may co-occur with communication disorders (e.g., feeding and swallowing problems, seizures, sensory impairments).					
79. Challenging behavior as a potential communication act.	Formalize the consideration of challenging behavior when developing behavioral assessments and interventions.	The communicative force of challenging behavior is recognized, but development of behavioral assessments and interventions doesn't officially involve SLPs.	Contact team psychologists for assistance in effecting change. Make other contacts based on result.	Communication Services Director	1 Start now.
80. Designing and working with a variety of service delivery models (e.g., classroom-based, pull-out, collaborative).					

A. Knowledge

Collectively, the team's knowledge supports and encourages communication. At least one team member has knowledge about:	Desired Change/Goals	Barriers and Resources	Action Needed	Who	Priority/ When
81. Family dynamics and the impact of severe disability on the family.					
82. The importance of incorporating current research findings into assessment and program implementation.					

> Time constraints and lack of a forum prevent staff members from sharing and discussing current research findings from the literature. The team, however, did not identify these issues as a priority to be addressed in this Action Plan.

Example #1 / Action Plan Section III   CSC   139

B. Skills and Experience

Team members' skills, experiences, and access to resources support and encourage communication. At least one team member has demonstrated the expertise or has the help of resource people who know how to:	Desired Change/Goals	Barriers and Resources	Action Needed	Who	Priority/When
83. Integrate the domains of cognitive, motor, sensory, and social functioning in communication *assessment* and *goal setting*.					
84. Integrate the domains of cognitive, motor, sensory, and social functioning in communication *implementation*.					
85. Provide ongoing assessment and evaluation using standardized and nonstandardized (formal or informal) procedures.	"Ongoing" is the troublesome word here. Our target is more involvement of SLPs on an ongoing basis.	Direct services providers are able to assess on an ongoing basis. Involvement of staff and significant others is critical, but leadership from SLPs is also needed.	SLPs will have more direct involvement in person-centered planning—see #16.	SLPs & QDDP	1 / Start now.
86. Plan and implement communication assessments that lead directly to functional communication intervention goals and objectives.	Improve communication skills aspect of person-centered planning.	Shortage of SLPs	SLPs will be more involved in person-centered planning.	SLPs	1 / Start now.

Communication Supports Checklist • McCarthy et al. • © 1998 Paul H. Brookes Publishing Co., Inc., Baltimore

B. Skills and Experience

Team members' skills, experiences, and access to resources support and encourage communication. At least one team member has demonstrated the expertise or has the help of resource people who know how to:

	Desired Change/Goals	Barriers and Resources	Action Needed	Who	Priority/When
87. Describe and document functional communication abilities and needs within specific contexts (e.g., educational settings, living environments, recreational environments, vocational environments, the community at large).					
88. Plan, implement, monitor, and modify, as needed, intervention programs that allow individuals to develop functional communication skills in spoken or AAC modes appropriate to educational, living, recreational, and work environments.					
89. Assess emergent and functional literacy skills across all environments.					
90. Teach emergent and functional literacy skills across all environments.					

The team reported that the integration of AAC across settings could be improved. SLPs will be able to address this issue as they work with other staff during direct services provision (see #9).

Communication Supports Checklist • McCarthy et al. • © 1998 Paul H. Brookes Publishing Co., Inc., Baltimore

Example #1 / Action Plan Section III   CSC   141

B. Skills and Experience

Team members' skills, experiences, and access to resources support and encourage communication. At least one team member has demonstrated the expertise or has the help of resource people who know how to:	Desired Change/Goals	Barriers and Resources	Action Needed	Who	Priority/When
91. Help the individual use the most appropriate (and least intrusive) positioning and mobility aids to maximize functional communication across a variety of environments.					
92. Manage activities of daily living and incorporate functional communication into each of these activities.					
93. Integrate cognition; oral and written communication; and motor, sensory, and social development in defining and implementing communication goals.					
94. Incorporate current research findings into assessment and program implementation.					

> Improvement in this area will probably occur as staff adjust to person-centered planning, which focuses on daily activities instead of isolated, out-of-context training sessions.

Communication Supports Checklist • McCarthy et al. • © 1998 Paul H. Brookes Publishing Co., Inc., Baltimore

B. Skills and Experience

(continued)

Team members' skills, experiences, and access to resources support and encourage communication. At least one team member has demonstrated the expertise or has the help of resource people who know how to:	Desired Change/Goals	Barriers and Resources	Action Needed	Who	Priority/When
95. Promote team participation and self-advocacy on the part of individuals with severe disabilities.					
96. Interact in a culturally sensitive manner.					
97. Understand laws that protect the rights of people with severe disabilities.					

> Team members noted that consideration of cultural values and traditions occasionally gets overlooked when working with individuals who have been at Sundale for a long time. The team, however, did not identify this issue as a high priority at this time.

Example #2

A Metropolitan School

Members of one school district's AAC and AT team completed the following Checklist and Action Plan. The team is based at North Hill School, a school for students with disabilities that is located in a large metropolitan area on the East Coast. North Hill is attended by 120 students from 4 to 21 years of age, all of whom receive services from the team. The students have sensory impairments; severe communication disorders; developmental disabilities such as autism, mental retardation, and cerebral palsy; and/or multiple physical disabilities. Each student uses some form of AAC or AT.

The team, which includes an OT, a nurse, a parent, SLPs, and a teacher, has been working at the school for more than 8 years. One of few in its area, the team serves as a model for similar teams and often receives visits from local education officials, government representatives, and the media.

Example #2   CSC   145

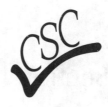

Communication Supports Checklist

For Programs Serving Individuals with Severe Disabilities

Check one: ☐ Individual member rating ☑ Team consensus rating

Program(s) and/or setting(s) evaluated:

North Hill School

Date:

January 15, 1998

Checklist completed by (list individual rater or team members and their roles/disciplines):

Sue Turner, O.T.R./L.

Michael Gomez, parent

Sam Blake, classroom teacher

Jake McCarthy, school nurse

Ken Simons, SLP

Jennifer Chang, SLP

Anna Green, SLP

Communication Supports Checklis: • McCarthy et al. • © 1998 Paul H. Brookes Publishing Co., Inc., Baltimore

Example #2 / Checklist   CSC   147

Section I

Overall Program Support for Communication

Instructions for Rating Items in this Section

When evaluating the program's Overall Program Support for Communication, your team should consider how much program policies, decisions, and practices reflect the values, attitudes, and beliefs listed in Parts A, B, and C of this section. Consider the program's written policies and routine practices as you evaluate these items. A rating of **Consistently True** means that this indicator is true of the attitudes and practices of virtually everyone who interacts with individuals served by the program. A rating of **Sometimes True** should be assigned if you feel that many (but not all) of the staff practices and agency policies are consistent with the attitude or belief identified in an item. A rating of **Rarely True** indicates that a particular attitude or value is rarely or never reflected in the program's routine policies and practices with individuals who have severe disabilities.

A. Philosophy

The following values, attitudes, and beliefs about communication are desirable in all decisions and interactions with individuals with severe disabilities. As a team, we behave in ways that reflect these beliefs:

	Consistently True	Sometimes True	Rarely True	COMMENTS
1. Communication is a basic human right.	✓			
2. All individuals should have opportunities to participate fully in their community.		✓		*During some special activities, staff do not include all students because of difficulties modifying the event and/or the environment.*
3. All individuals should have freedom of action and choice.	✓			
4. All individuals communicate in some way; communication may be nonspoken, nonsymbolic, and/or nonintentional.	✓			

Communication Supports Checklist • McCarthy et al. • © 1998 Paul H. Brookes Publishing Co., Inc., Baltimore

Example #2 / Checklist Section I   CSC   149

A.   Philosophy

The following values, attitudes, and beliefs about communication are desirable in all decisions and interactions with individuals with severe disabilities. As a team, we behave in ways that reflect these beliefs:

	Consistently True	Sometimes True	Rarely True	COMMENTS
5. Appropriate communication goals improve quality of life.	✔			
6. Individuals with severe disabilities and their primary communication partners are involved in communication goal setting and intervention.	✔			
7. Individual and family choices are respected.	✔			
8. Diverse family values and traditions are recognized and respected.		✔		*Some staff members aren't always aware that a student's response is rooted in his or her cultural or religious background.*

Communication Supports Checklist • McCarthy et al. • © 1998 Paul H. Brookes Publishing Co., Inc., Baltimore

A. Philosophy

The following values, attitudes, and beliefs about communication are desirable in all decisions and interactions with individuals with severe disabilities. As a team, we behave in ways that reflect these beliefs:

	Consistently True	Sometimes True	Rarely True	COMMENTS
9. Team collaboration is essential for effective service.	✓			*Some paraprofessionals have changed positioning & switch placement options before consulting professional staff.*

Example #2 / Checklist Section I   CSC   151

B. Protection of Communication Rights

The program ensures the basic communication rights of individuals, regardless of the nature or severity of their disabilities. In the settings being inventoried, communication partners:	Consistently True	Sometimes True	Rarely True	COMMENTS
10. Recognize and acknowledge initiations for social interactions.	✓			
11. Recognize and acknowledge requests (for objects, actions, events, people, information, and feedback).	✓			
12. Recognize and acknowledge expressions of feelings and attitudes.	✓			
13. Honor preferences indicated by individuals.	✓			

Communication Supports Checklist • McCarthy et al. • © 1998 Paul H. Brookes Publishing Co., Inc., Baltimore

B.   Protection of Communication Rights

(continued)

The program ensures the basic communication rights of individuals, regardless of the nature or severity of their disabilities. In the settings being inventoried, communication partners:	Consistently True	Sometimes True	Rarely True	COMMENTS
14. Offer multiple choices in activities throughout the day.			✓	*Occurs when a member of the AAC team or therapy dept. is primary communication partner. Two of eleven classroom teachers offer choices.*
15. Acknowledge and honor rejections unless the undesired action, event, or object is essential to the individual's protection from harm.	✓			
16. Arrange comprehensive communication assessments and individually appropriate interventions for individuals who might benefit from communication intervention services, regardless of age and severity of disability.	✓			*Identification of need & recommendation for evaluation most often come from team or therapy staff. Occasionally referral comes from teacher, administrator, or parent.*
17. Include peers without disabilities who convey respect and courtesy.		✓		*We have a relationship with neighboring elementary and middle schools for community field trips. Team members and therapy staff generally attend.*

Communication Supports Checklist • McCarthy et al. • © 1998 Paul H. Brookes Publishing Co., Inc., Baltimore

Example #2 / Checklist Section I   CSC   153

B. Protection of Communication Rights

The program ensures the basic communication rights of individuals, regardless of the nature or severity of their disabilities. In the settings being inventoried, communication partners:

	Consistently True	Sometimes True	Rarely True	COMMENTS
18. Do not discuss an individual in the third person when that individual is present.	✓			
19. Ensure that individuals have access to assistive technology (AT), augmentative and alternative communication (AAC) devices, and support systems needed for communication at all times.	✓			*Occurs primarily if team members or therapy staff are involved. Special area teachers (music, art, & gym teachers) have also increased their active involvement in utilizing AAC.*
20. Ensure that AT and AAC devices are in good working order at all times.	✓			
21. Offer information and explanations when appropriate (e.g., introductions to a classroom or jobsite visitor, explanation about the need to change a planned activity).	✓			*Our school has a large number of visitors, including educators, government officials, & the media. Our administrator often finds team members, therapy staff, or specific classroom teachers to provide demonstrations or explanations.*

Communication Supports Checklist • McCarthy et al. • © 1998 Paul H. Brookes Publishing Co., Inc., Baltimore

C. Environmental Support for Communication

CSC

The environments in which people learn, live, play, and work should promote and support communication. People in each of our program's settings do so by:	Consistently True	Sometimes True	Rarely True	COMMENTS
22. Expecting communication (e.g., waiting for an initiation or a response, maintaining visual contact).	✓			
23. Providing interesting and age-appropriate materials, communication partners, and activities.	✓			Team members and therapy staff set up interactive communication activities at jobsite, in the classroom, & in the community. Otherwise, students are most typically "herded" through the activity.
24. Following policies and practices that do not prohibit or restrict communication.	✓			
25. Including communication partners who know how to use AAC systems and devices used by individuals (e.g., American Sign Language, graphic symbols, high- and low-technology devices).	✓			

Communication Supports Checklist • McCarthy et al. • © 1998 Paul H. Brookes Publishing Co., Inc., Baltimore

Example #2 / Checklist Section I   CSC   155

C. Environmental Support for Communication *(continued)*

The environments in which people learn, live, play, and work should promote and support communication. People in each of our program's settings do so by:	Consistently True	Sometimes True	Rarely True	COMMENTS
26. Arranging materials so individuals without symbolic communication skills can indicate their interests or requests through the use of gaze, natural gestures, and/or vocal or behavioral signals.			✓	*We need to review the research literature on this topic and determine how we can arrange the environment and materials to foster communication.*
27. Including peers without disabilities who are available for communication interactions.		✓		
28. Including communication partners who use appropriate language (e.g., primary language) and appropriate communication mode(s) (e.g., oral, signed, graphic, adapted for vision or hearing impairments).	✓			

Communication Supports Checklist • McCarthy et al. • © 1998 Paul H. Brookes Publishing Co., Inc., Baltimore

Section II

Assessment Practices, Goal-Setting Practices, and Program Implementation

---

Instructions for Rating Items in this Section

When evaluating the program's Assessment Practices, Goal-Setting Practices, and Program Implementation, your team should consider whether and how much the program's actual practices are consistent with the ideal practices identified in Parts A, B, and C of this section. Consider the program's written procedural policies and routine practices as you consider these items. When rating each item, a rating of **Consistently True** means the statement is consistently true of the practices used by all people involved in communication assessment, goal setting, and program implementation. A rating of **Sometimes True** might indicate some efforts to adopt the practices in the program or that one or two staff members in the program do use the practices. A rating of **Rarely True** indicates that a particular practice is rarely or never reflected in the way that communication needs and abilities are assessed, the way that goals are established, and/or the way that a program is implemented for individuals with severe disabilities served by your program.

Example #2 / Checklist Section II   CSC   157

A.   Assessment Practices

CSC

Communication interactions should be observed carefully before program implementation is designed. The degree to which settings are sensitive and responsive to each person's communication needs should also be observed. Goals can be chosen for individuals and the places where they learn, live, play, and work. When assessing an individual's communication abilities and needs, team members:	Consistently True	Sometimes True	Rarely True	COMMENTS
29. Describe the individual's current communication modes (including intentional, nonintentional, symbolic, and non-symbolic communication).	✓			*It is often difficult to determine when challenging behavior has a communicative intent.*
30. Include measures of sensory responsivity (i.e., hearing and vision tests) by appropriate professionals.	✓			
31. Include measures of physical status (e.g., positioning, sensorimotor, joint range of motion, motor control) by appropriate professionals.	✓			
32. Identify social functions (e.g., comment, protest, request) of communication behavior across settings.	✓			

A. Assessment Practices

(continued)

Communication interactions should be observed carefully before program implementation is designed. The degree to which settings are sensitive and responsive to each person's communication needs should also be observed. Goals can be chosen for individuals and the places where they learn, live, play, and work. When assessing an individual's communication abilities and needs, team members:

	Consistently True	Sometimes True	Rarely True	COMMENTS
33. Identify the individual's primary communication partners.	✔			
34. Conduct multiple observations over time.	✔			*This is always considered but is not always formally written in assessment reports.*
35. Measure the responsiveness of partners to communication acts.		✔		
36. Measure opportunities for communication across environments (e.g., education, living, leisure, work).	✔			

Example #2 / Checklist Section II   CSC   159

A. Assessment Practices
(continued)

Communication interactions should be observed carefully before program implementation is designed. The degree to which settings are sensitive and responsive to each person's communication needs should also be observed. Goals can be chosen for individuals and the places where they learn, live, play, and work. When assessing an individual's communication abilities and needs, team members:

	Consistently True	Sometimes True	Rarely True	COMMENTS
37. Identify the specific communication forms and uses in various modes (e.g., speech, writing, AAC) that are useful across settings.	✔			
38. Measure the spontaneity of communication.	✔			*A student with a communication disability or an advocate is not always involved in team meetings.*
39. Use a team model that includes the individual, family members, peers, friends, professionals, support personnel, and other significant communication partners.	✔			
40. Specifically ask family members to provide information about perceived communication needs.	✔			

Communication Supports Checklist • McCarthy et al. • © 1998 Paul H. Brookes Publishing Co., Inc., Baltimore

A. Assessment Practices

(continued)

Communication interactions should be observed carefully before program implementation is designed. The degree to which settings are sensitive and responsive to each person's communication needs should also be observed. Goals can be chosen for individuals and the places where they learn, live, play, and work. When assessing an individual's communication abilities and needs, team members:

	Consistently True	Sometimes True	Rarely True	COMMENTS
41. Provide explanations of assessment procedures and results in ways that are meaningful to all team members, including the individual with severe disabilities.	✓			
42. Provide information about communication needs that partners notice during their activities and interactions with individuals.		✓		*Paraprofessionals should share information with other team members about communication events that occur regularly.*

B. Goal-Setting Practices

When reaching consensus on appropriate and attainable program implementation goals for an individual, the team:	Consistently True	Sometimes True	Rarely True	COMMENTS
43. Selects and prioritizes goals based on their importance and potential impact on an individual's quality of life.	✔			*While writing initial assessment reports, team members do prioritize goals. Classroom teachers may or may not consider quality-of-life priorities when IEPs are written.*
44. Uses a team model that includes the individual as well as family members, peers, friends, professionals, support personnel, and other significant communication partners during the planning and implementation of communication interventions.		✔		*Students with communication disabilities don't always participate actively in goal setting.*
45. Considers environmental as well as individual goals.		✔		*Sometimes the environment isn't evaluated or modified to support students' communication.*
46. Takes into account an individual's existing intentional (e.g., pointing to a picture display) and/or nonintentional (e.g., crying) communication abilities.	✔			

B.   Goal-Setting Practices

When reaching consensus on appropriate and attainable program implementation goals for an individual, the team:	Consistently True	Sometimes True	Rarely True	COMMENTS
47. Selects goals consistent with a logical hierarchy of skills and identifies short-term objectives that seem realistically attainable for an individual within a specified time frame (e.g., 6 months, 1 year).	✔			
48. Selects short-term objectives that are consistent with the long-term goals for an individual.	✔			
49. Selects goals that will support an individual's transition to a new environment (e.g., from school to work).		✔		
50. Reviews information from previous teams to ensure continuity of an individual's goals (e.g., person worked on two-choice picture-pointing skills in previous program as a step toward use of a more complex communication board. In new program, team agrees to move on to three-choice picture board).	✔			

C. Program Implementation

Program implementation is based on assessment and selected functional communication goals across settings. Ongoing evaluation is used to measure outcomes and adjust practices accordingly. When implementing intervention programs, the team:

	Consistently True	Sometimes True	Rarely True	COMMENTS
51. Targets communication goals primarily in an individual's natural environments during typical interactions, rather than in isolated environments.	✔			*Carryover of goals in this whole section when a team member is not the facilitator is entirely dependent on the motivation level of the classroom teacher (who is also the case manager).*
52. Uses pull-out intervention only when necessary for additional practice.	✔			*Occurs when parents insist; a decision to use pull-out intervention isn't always based on student needs. Sometimes pull-out intervention is not built into the student's IEP, even when it is needed.*
53. Provides opportunities for initiation, maintenance, and termination of communication/social interactions.	✔			
54. Provides opportunities to communicate across all environments.	✔			

Communication Supports Checklist • McCarthy et al. • © 1998 Paul H. Brookes Publishing Co., Inc., Baltimore

C. Program Implementation

Program implementation is based on assessment and selected functional communication goals across settings. Ongoing evaluation is used to measure outcomes and adjust practices accordingly. When implementing intervention programs, the team:

	Consistently True	Sometimes True	Rarely True	COMMENTS
55. Uses an individual's current communication systems while promoting new skill acquisition.	✓			
56. Uses communication supports and systems that are appropriate to each individual's physical abilities.	✓			
57. Uses communication supports and systems that are appropriate to each individual's sensory abilities.	✓			
58. Uses communication supports and systems that are appropriate to each individual's cognitive abilities.		✓		*Some staff believe that prerequisite cognitive skills are needed before introducing an AAC system.*

Example #2 / Checklist Section II   CSC   165

C. Program Implementation

(continued)

Program implementation is based on assessment and selected functional communication goals across settings. Ongoing evaluation is used to measure outcomes and adjust practices accordingly. When implementing intervention programs, the team:

	Consistently True	Sometimes True	Rarely True	COMMENTS
59. Uses communication supports and systems that are appropriate to each individual's communication needs and environments across settings.	✔			*See #51.*
60. Includes necessary adaptations or modifications to the environment to optimize an individual's use of communication supports and systems (e.g., mounting AAC device on wheelchair).	✔			
61. Provides for the seating and positioning needs of individuals who use communication supports and systems.	✔			*We could provide more ergonomically supportive chairs.*
62. Makes assistive devices available to help individuals use supports for communication (e.g., hand/wrist splint, head-controlled pointer, control switches).	✔			

C. Program Implementation

Program implementation is based on assessment and selected functional communication goals across settings. Ongoing evaluation is used to measure outcomes and adjust practices accordingly. When implementing intervention programs, the team:	Consistently True	Sometimes True	Rarely True	COMMENTS
63. Integrates elements of individual instruction by all team members involved.	✔			
64. Implements plans as designed to accomplish stated goals.	✔			
65. Uses a team model that includes the individual, family members, friends, peers, professionals, support personnel, and other significant communication partners.	✔			*During implementation, we include family members, advocates, an audiologist, a physician, a PT, an OT, a psychologist, an SLP, a classroom teacher, and a special education teacher.*
66. Builds on goals and strategies developed in previous programs.	✔			

Example #2 / Checklist Section II   CSC   167

C. Program Implementation

(continued)

Program implementation is based on assessment and selected functional communication goals across settings. Ongoing evaluation is used to measure outcomes and adjust practices accordingly. When implementing intervention programs, the team:

	Consistently True	Sometimes True	Rarely True	COMMENTS
67. Includes and implements plans for continuity and transfer of information regarding communication supports and services before an individual changes program placement.	✔			*A team member does not always attend transition-planning meetings.*
68. Includes a specific time schedule for team reassessment of all program elements.	✔			*Follow-up meetings are often canceled when issues that seem more important come up.*

Section III

Team Competencies

Instructions for Rating Items in this Section

Rate the knowledge and skills that team members contribute as combined resources. Specific types of knowledge and skills are identified in Parts A and B of this section. Consider the specific training, experiences, and expertise of each team member, including family members, as you consider these items. When rating these items, a rating of **Consistently True** means that one or more team members has outstanding knowledge, skills, and/or experience relevant to that particular item. A rating of **Sometimes True** should be assigned if you believe that one or two (but not all) team members demonstrate this knowledge or skill. A rating of **Sometimes True** should also be assigned if you have the occasional help of a resource person (not a regular member of the team), but the team agrees that it would be desirable for additional team members to share this knowledge or skill or that the levels of expertise could be improved. A rating of **Rarely True** indicates that a particular knowledge or skill is clearly not demonstrated by any single member of the team.

Example #2 / Checklist Section III   CSC   169

A. Knowledge

Collectively, the team's knowledge supports and encourages communication. At least one team member has knowledge about:	Consistently True	Sometimes True	Rarely True	COMMENTS
69. Human development.	✓			
70. Communication development, including reading and writing.		✓		*SLPs have knowledge of communication development, but this is not always the case with teachers and other team members.*
71. Individuals with severe disabilities across ages and levels of independence.	✓			
72. Factors that prevent secondary conditions that interfere with communication (e.g., swallowing disorders, poor positioning, challenging behavior).	✓			

Communication Supports Checklist • McCarthy et al. • © 1998 Paul H. Brookes Publishing Co., Inc., Baltimore

A. Knowledge

Collectively, the team's knowledge supports and encourages communication. At least one team member has knowledge about:

	Consistently True	Sometimes True	Rarely True	COMMENTS
73. Different means of communication (e.g., body posture, vocalization, gaze, gesture, sign language, electronic and nonelectronic systems).	✓			
74. Different types of communication symbols (e.g., pictures, braille, words, signs, speech).		✓		*Again, some staff members have little knowledge of symbol systems.*
75. Amplification and other AT useful to people who have severe disabilities with accompanying sensory limitations.	✓			
76. Medications and their effects on behavior, especially communication.		✓		*We consult with the school nurse & pediatrician.*

Communication Supports Checklist • McCarthy et al. • © 1998 Paul H. Brookes Publishing Co., Inc., Baltimore

Example #2 / Checklist Section III   CSC   171

A. Knowledge

Collectively, the team's knowledge supports and encourages communication. At least one team member has knowledge about:	Consistently True	Sometimes True	Rarely True	COMMENTS
77. Motor control, muscle tone, and positioning as these affect communication.	✓			*OT and PT staff are consulted regularly.*
78. Disabilities that may co-occur with communication disorders (e.g., feeding and swallowing problems, seizures, sensory impairments).	✓			
79. Challenging behavior as a potential communication act.	✓			
80. Designing and working with a variety of service delivery models (e.g., classroom-based, pull-out, collaborative).	✓			

Communication Supports Checklist • McCarthy et al. • © 1998 Paul H. Brookes Publishing Co., Inc., Baltimore

A. Knowledge

Collectively, the team's knowledge supports and encourages communication. At least one team member has knowledge about:	Consistently True	Sometimes True	Rarely True	COMMENTS
81. Family dynamics and the impact of severe disability on the family.	✔			We need to make a concerted effort to read the current research literature on this topic and share new ideas and information.
82. The importance of incorporating current research findings into assessment and program implementation.		✔		With everything else we have to do, it's hard to keep up with current research!

Communication Supports Checklist • McCarthy et al. • © 1998 Paul H. Brookes Publishing Co., Inc., Baltimore

Example #2 / Checklist Section III   CSC   173

B.   Skills and Experience

Team members' skills, experiences, and access to resources support and encourage communication. At least one team member has demonstrated the expertise or has the help of resource people who know how to:

	Consistently True	Sometimes True	Rarely True	COMMENTS
83. Integrate the domains of cognitive, motor, sensory, and social functioning in communication *assessment* and *goal setting*.	✔			
84. Integrate the domains of cognitive, motor, sensory, and social functioning in communication *implementation*.	✔			
85. Provide ongoing assessment and evaluation using standardized and nonstandardized (formal or informal) procedures.		✔		*We all have trouble getting consistent and reliable information on spontaneous communication use in natural settings.*
86. Plan and implement communication assessments that lead directly to functional communication intervention goals and objectives.	✔			

Communication Supports Checklist • McCarthy et al. • © 1998 Paul H. Brookes Publishing Co., Inc., Baltimore

B.   Skills and Experience

Team members' skills, experiences, and access to resources support and encourage communication. At least one team member has demonstrated the expertise or has the help of resource people who know how to:

	Consistently True	Sometimes True	Rarely True	COMMENTS
87. Describe and document functional communication abilities and needs within specific contexts (e.g., educational settings, living environments, recreational environments, vocational environments, the community at large).		✓		*We can't really say we are able to do this—scheduling constraints do not permit observations in some settings outside school, such as living environments.*
88. Plan, implement, monitor, and modify, as needed, intervention programs that allow individuals to develop functional communication skills in spoken or AAC modes appropriate to educational, living, recreational, and work environments.	✓			
89. Assess emergent and functional literacy skills across all environments.	✓			
90. Teach emergent and functional literacy skills across all environments.	✓			

Communication Supports Checklist • McCarthy et al. • © 1998 Paul H. Brookes Publishing Co., Inc., Baltimore

Example #2 / Checklist Section III   CSC   175

B.   Skills and Experience *(continued)*

Team members' skills, experiences, and access to resources support and encourage communication. At least one team member has demonstrated the expertise or has the help of resource people who know how to:	Consistently True	Sometimes True	Rarely True	COMMENTS
91. Help the individual use the most appropriate (and least intrusive) positioning and mobility aids to maximize functional communication across a variety of environments.	✔			
92. Manage activities of daily living and incorporate functional communication into each of these activities.		✔		*We have expertise in managing activities of daily living (teachers) and functional communication (AAC staff), but these areas aren't consistently integrated.*
93. Integrate cognition; oral and written communication; and motor, sensory, and social development in defining and implementing communication goals.	✔			
94. Incorporate current research findings into assessment and program implementation.		✔		*Again, we realize that this is important, but it's hard to find time to incorporate current research findings!*

B.   Skills and Experience

Team members' skills, experiences, and access to resources support and encourage communication. At least one team member has demonstrated the expertise or has the help of resource people who know how to:

	Consistently True	Sometimes True	Rarely True	COMMENTS
95. Promote team participation and self-advocacy on the part of individuals with severe disabilities.	✔			*We haven't found a way to make participation truly meaningful for students with more severe disabilities.*
96. Interact in a culturally sensitive manner.	✔			
97. Understand laws that protect the rights of people with severe disabilities.	✔			

Example #2 / Checklist Section III   CSC   177

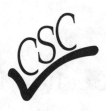

Communication Supports Action Plan

For Programs Serving Individuals with Severe Disabilities

Date Checklist (team consensus rating) completed:

January 15, 1998

Date Action Plan completed:

January 22, 1998

Action Plan completed by (list team members and their roles/disciplines):

Ken Simons, SLP

Jennifer Chang, SLP

Anna Green, SLP

Michael Gomez, parent

Sue Turner, O.T.R./L.

Sam Blake, classroom teacher

Jake McCarthy, school nurse

Communication Supports Checklist • McCarthy et al. • © 1998 Paul H. Brookes Publishing Co., Inc., Baltimore

Example #2 / Action Plan   CSC   179

Section I

Overall Program Support for Communication

A. Philosophy

The following values, attitudes, and beliefs about communication are desirable in all decisions and interactions with individuals with severe disabilities. As a team, we behave in ways that reflect these beliefs:

	Desired Change/Goals	Barriers and Resources	Action Needed	Who	Priority/When
1. Communication is a basic human right.					
2. All individuals should have opportunities to participate fully in their community.	All students should be included in school activities whenever possible.	Desire and ability of staff to make special arrangements to include students	Consult with OT to find ways to modify environment.	Teachers and OT	2 Before scheduled special activities
3. All individuals should have freedom of action and choice.					
4. All individuals communicate in some way; communication may be nonspoken, nonsymbolic, and/or nonintentional.					

A. Philosophy

The following values, attitudes, and beliefs about communication are desirable in all decisions and interactions with individuals with severe disabilities. As a team, we behave in ways that reflect these beliefs:	Desired Change/Goals	Barriers and Resources	Action Needed	Who	Priority/When
5. Appropriate communication goals improve quality of life.					
6. Individuals with severe disabilities and their primary communication partners are involved in communication goal setting and intervention.					
7. Individual and family choices are respected.					
8. Diverse family values and traditions are recognized and respected.	*Increase staff awareness of different cultural and religious traditions.*	*Need time in schedule*	*In-service training for staff on different cultural traditions*	*SLPs, AAC staff*	*2* *Before next school year*

Communication Supports Checklist • McCarthy et al. • © 1998 Paul H. Brookes Publishing Co., Inc., Baltimore

A. Philosophy

The following values, attitudes, and beliefs about communication are desirable in all decisions and interactions with individuals with severe disabilities. As a team, we behave in ways that reflect these beliefs:

	Desired Change/Goals	Barriers and Resources	Action Needed	Who	Priority/When
9. Team collaboration is essential for effective service.	Students will receive new positions for access or various opportunities for access with collaboration of professionals and paraprofessionals.	Paraprofessional's frustration in wanting child to succeed immediately & time pressures of coordination with therapy staff	Monthly formal meetings between classroom (paraprofessional) staff and therapy staff	SLPs & teachers	1 Already started

> The team noted that sometimes paraprofessionals adjusted positioning and switch placement before consulting with professional staff members.

B.   Protection of Communication Rights

The program ensures the basic communication rights of individuals, regardless of the nature or severity of their disabilities. In the settings being inventoried, communication partners:	Desired Change/Goals	Barriers and Resources	Action Needed	Who		Priority/When
10. Recognize and acknowledge initiations for social interactions.	Add objective to students' IEPs: to have opportunities for initiating or indicating desire for interaction.	Teachers' desire and awareness are needed for these opportunities to occur.	Set up specific time for teacher to interact with student in a manageable setting in which attention getting is appropriate.	AAC staff	1	At annual review meeting
11. Recognize and acknowledge requests (for objects, actions, events, people, information, and feedback).	Add objective to students' IEPs: to have opportunity to request.	See #10.	Either set up specific times in day for this to occur, or determine opportunities for requesting within each part of school day (opening, transition to jobsite, elective class, etc.).	SLPs to help classroom teachers plan	1	At annual review
12. Recognize and acknowledge expressions of feelings and attitudes.	Add objective to students' IEPs: to have opportunities to comment.	See #10.	Determine opportunities for commenting within each part of school day (opening, transition to jobsite, elective class, etc.)	SLPs to help classroom teachers plan	1	Meet weekly or biweekly to plan.
13. Honor preferences indicated by individuals.						

> Over the past 3 years, the team has attempted to meet with classroom teachers to plan how to meet these goals. Teachers have reported lack of time to meet or haven't always implemented suggestions on a regular basis.

Communication Supports Checklist • McCarthy et al. • © 1998 Paul H. Brookes Publishing Co., Inc., Baltimore

B.   Protection of Communication Rights   *(continued)*

The program ensures the basic communication rights of individuals, regardless of the nature or severity of their disabilities. In the settings being inventoried, communication partners:

	Desired Change/Goals	Barriers and Resources	Action Needed	Who		Priority/ When
14. Offer multiple choices in activities throughout the day.	Add objective to students' IEPs: to have opportunities to make choices.	Teachers' desire and awareness are needed.	Determine opportunities for commenting within each part of school day (opening, transition to jobsite, elective class, etc.).	SLPs to help classroom teachers plan	1	Meet weekly or bi-weekly to plan.
15. Acknowledge and honor rejections unless the undesired action, event, or object is essential to the individual's protection from harm.						
16. Arrange comprehensive communication assessments and individually appropriate interventions for individuals who might benefit from communication intervention services, regardless of age and severity of disability.	At all annual reviews, any student currently not receiving AAC services will be assessed.	Case managers (teachers) need reminders regarding referral process.	Review case management responsibilities & procedures in memo, & bring up at staff meetings.	Administrator, guidance counselor	3	During next school year
17. Include peers without disabilities who convey respect and courtesy.	Identify this concern at faculty meetings & staff retreat.	Time to discuss this issue during meetings and retreat	Formal announcement listed on meeting agenda	Administrator	1	At _next_ meeting and retreat

> The team noted that therapy staff made recommendations for assessment more often than teachers, administrators, or parents.

Communication Supports Checklist • McCarthy et al. • © 1998 Paul H. Brookes Publishing Co., Inc., Baltimore

Example #2 / Action Plan Section I   CSC   185

B. Protection of Communication Rights *(continued)*

The program ensures the basic communication rights of individuals, regardless of the nature or severity of their disabilities. In the settings being inventoried, communication partners:	Desired Change/Goals	Barriers and Resources	Action Needed	Who	Priority/When
18. Do not discuss an individual in the third person when that individual is present.	Staff will not "talk around" students (formally or informally) when students are present.	Lack of awareness of policy	Review policy of no "talking around" students in faculty meeting and administrative memo.	Administrator	2 — By start of next school year
19. Ensure that individuals have access to assistive technology (AT), augmentative and alternative communication (AAC) devices, and support systems needed for communication at all times.	Workshops for support staff regarding the need for access to AAC devices (Teachers will receive this info as needed: "Please bring Michael's AAC equipment on field trip.")	Time during school hours when paraprofessionals can leave classrooms for workshops with SLPs	Provide workshops during school hours. Arrange for special area teachers (music, gym, art) to work with students while paraprofessionals are in workshops.	AAC team, administrators	2 — Plan before next school year.
20. Ensure that AT and AAC devices are in good working order at all times.	During classroom morning routine staff members or peers should check AAC devices by greeting students who use AAC.	Time in schedule, identification of responsible party	Establish routine in a planning session.	SLPs & teachers	2 — By start of next school year
21. Offer information and explanations when appropriate (e.g., introductions to a classroom or jobsite visitor, explanation about the need to change a planned activity).					

C. Environmental Support for Communication

The environments in which people learn, live, play, and work should promote and support communication. People in each of our program's settings do so by:

	Desired Change/Goals	Barriers and Resources	Action Needed	Who	Priority/When
22. Expecting communication (e.g., waiting for an initiation or a response, maintaining visual contact).	SLP to continue modeling communication facilitation techniques (especially waiting for responses) during therapy sessions, community trips, & class lessons.	Lack of staff knowledge	SLP modeling will continue. Also, SLPs will give staff members positive reinforcement: "That was great, you waited for Sandi to answer!"	SLPs	1 — Ongoing
23. Providing interesting and age-appropriate materials, communication partners, and activities.	Encourage meaningful participation rather than passive participation during activities.	Participation should be encouraged even when SLPs aren't present.	Develop weekly logs for staff to list purposeful student communication observed in a variety of settings.	SLPs, teachers	2 — Suggest at spring retreat.
24. Following policies and practices that do not prohibit or restrict communication.					
25. Including communication partners who know how to use AAC systems and devices used by individuals (e.g., American Sign Language, graphic symbols, high- and low-technology devices).	In-service training on the importance of AAC will be provided—see #19. Also, maintain inclusion opportunities by continuing joint field trips and activities with other schools.	Funding, willingness of other schools' staff to participate	Have activity in mind; contact interested staff member at other school for planning.	SLPs, teachers	3 — Ongoing

The team found that students were sometimes "herded" through activities.

Communication Supports Checklist • McCarthy et al. • © 1998 Paul H. Brookes Publishing Co., Inc., Baltimore

Example #2 / Action Plan Section I   CSC   187

C. Environmental Support for Communication

The environments in which people learn, live, play, and work should promote and support communication. People in each of our program's settings do so by:	Desired Change/Goals	Barriers and Resources	Action Needed	Who	Priority/When
26. Arranging materials so individuals without symbolic communication skills can indicate their interests or requests through the use of gaze, natural gestures, and/or vocal or behavioral signals.	Reengineer classroom and worksite settings.	Time in schedules, willingness of teachers to participate & follow up	Hold planning meetings and work sessions to set up environment.	Teachers, SLPs, other team members	3 — By end of next year
27. Including peers without disabilities who are available for communication interactions.	Field trips with other schools will continue—see #25.			See #25.	
28. Including communication partners who use appropriate language (e.g., primary language) and appropriate communication mode(s) (e.g., oral, signed, graphic, adapted for vision or hearing impairments).					

> The team agreed that environments were rarely arranged for nonsymbolic communication to take place.

Communication Supports Checklist • McCarthy et al. • © 1998 Paul H. Brookes Publishing Co., Inc., Baltimore

Section II

Assessment Practices,
Goal-Setting Practices, and Program Implementation

Example #2 / Action Plan Section II   CSC   189

A. Assessment Practices

Communication interactions should be observed carefully before a program implementation is designed. The degree to which settings are sensitive and responsive to each person's communication needs should also be observed. Goals can be chosen for individuals and the places where they learn, live, play, and work. When assessing an individual's communication abilities and needs, team members:

	Desired Change/Goals	Barriers and Resources	Action Needed	Who	Priority/When
29. Describe the individual's current communication modes (including intentional, nonintentional, symbolic, and nonsymbolic communication).	Team members will become better at recognizing when challenging behavior serves as communication.	Sometimes staff members are frustrated with challenging behavior.	In-service training—SLPs to demonstrate multiple communicative purposes of challenging behavior.	SLPs and rest of team	1 · Spring in-service days
30. Include measures of sensory responsivity (i.e., hearing and vision tests) by appropriate professionals.					
31. Include measures of physical status (e.g., positioning, sensorimotor, joint range of motion, motor control) by appropriate professionals.					
32. Identify social functions (e.g., comment, protest, request) of communication behavior across settings.					

A. Assessment Practices

Communication interactions should be observed carefully before a program implementation is designed. The degree to which settings are sensitive and responsive to each person's communication needs should also be observed. Goals can be chosen for individuals and the places where they learn, live, play, and work. When assessing an individual's communication abilities and needs, team members:

	Desired Change/Goals	Barriers and Resources	Action Needed	Who	Priority/When
33. Identify the individual's primary communication partners.					
34. Conduct multiple observations over time.					
35. Measure the responsiveness of partners to communication acts.	During assessments, set up communication opportunities with a variety of partners.	Partners' responsiveness isn't a part of assessments.	Add to assessment protocol.	SLP	2 — By next assessment period
36. Measure opportunities for communication across environments (e.g., education, living, leisure, work).					

Communication Supports Checklist • McCarthy et al. • © 1998 Paul H. Brookes Publishing Co., Inc., Baltimore

Example #2 / Action Plan Section II   CSC   191

A.   Assessment Practices

Communication interactions should be observed carefully before a program implementation is designed. The degree to which settings are sensitive and responsive to each person's communication needs should also be observed. Goals can be chosen for individuals and the places where they learn, live, play, and work. When assessing an individual's communication abilities and needs, team members:

	Desired Change/Goals	Barriers and Resources	Action Needed	Who	Priority/When
37. Identify the specific communication forms and uses in various modes (e.g., speech, writing, AAC) that are useful across settings.					
38. Measure the spontaneity of communication.					
39. Use a team model that includes the individual, family members, peers, friends, professionals, support personnel, and other significant communication partners.	Involve students or family/ advocates in team meetings (IEP meetings, etc.).	Time constraints; greater understanding of the value of self-advocacy and self-determination	Schedule meetings when students can attend; provide needed communication supports. Provide info on self-advocacy, & discuss with staff.	Entire team	1	Begin at next team meeting.
40. Specifically ask family members to provide information about perceived communication needs.					

Communication Supports Checklist • McCarthy et al. • © 1998 Paul H. Brookes Publishing Co., Inc., Baltimore

A. Assessment Practices

Communication interactions should be observed carefully before a program implementation is designed. The degree to which settings are sensitive and responsive to each person's communication needs should also be observed. Goals can be chosen for individuals and the places where they learn, live, play, and work. When assessing an individual's communication abilities and needs, team members:

	Desired Change/Goals	Barriers and Resources	Action Needed	Who	Priority/When
41. Provide explanations of assessment procedures and results in a way that is meaningful to all team members, including the individual with severe disabilities.	Paraprofessionals will talk with other team members about communication interactions they have with students.	Paraprofessionals sometimes believe that their observations & opinions are unimportant; they also need more information about communication forms/modes.	Discuss value of paraprofessionals' contributions; hold in-service training about communication forms/ modes.	SLPs & other team members	2 · By next school year
42. Provide information about communication needs that partners notice during their activities and interactions with individuals.					

Communication Supports Checklist • McCarthy et al. • © 1998 Paul H. Brookes Publishing Co., Inc., Baltimore

Example #2 / Action Plan Section II   CSC   193

B. Goal-Setting Practices

When reaching consensus on appropriate and attainable program implementation goals for an individual, the team:	Desired Change/Goals	Barriers and Resources	Action Needed	Who	Priority/When
43. Selects and prioritizes goals based on their importance and potential impact on an individual's quality of life.					
44. Uses a team model that includes the individual as well as family members, peers, friends, professionals, support personnel, and other significant communication partners during the planning and implementation of communication interventions.	*Involve students with communication disabilities, parents, or advocates in goal setting.*	*We need a team facilitator who can make sure that students are included in meetings and that they participate actively.*	*Identify team member responsible for facilitating team meetings and involving all members.*	*Any team member*	*1* *By next team meeting*
45. Considers environmental as well as individual goals.					
46. Takes into account an individual's existing intentional (e.g., pointing to a picture display) and/or nonintentional (e.g., crying) communication abilities.					

B. Goal-Setting Practices

(continued)

When reaching consensus on appropriate and attainable program implementation goals for an individual, the team:	Desired Change/Goals	Barriers and Resources	Action Needed	Who	Priority/ When
47. Selects goals consistent with a logical hierarchy of skills and identifies short-term objectives that seem realistically attainable for an individual within a specified time frame (e.g., 6 months, 1 year).					
48. Selects short-term objectives that are consistent with the long-term goals for an individual.					
49. Selects goals that will support an individual's transition to a new environment (e.g., from school to work).	Team members should find out when transition meetings occur and ask to be included in the meetings.	Time in schedule for additional lengthy meetings	Get transition meeting agendas in advance, & come with suggestions for achieving goals.	SLP or other team member	1 / As transition meetings occur
50. Reviews information from previous teams to ensure continuity of an individual's goals (e.g., person worked on two-choice picture-pointing skills in previous program as a step toward use of a more complex communication board. In new program, team agrees to move on to three-choice picture board).					

The team noted that transition-planning meetings are not always attended by a team member.

Communication Supports Checklist • McCarthy et al. • © 1998 Paul H. Brookes Publishing Co., Inc., Baltimore

Example #2 / Action Plan Section II   CSC   195

C. Program Implementation

Program implementation is based on assessment and selected functional communication goals across settings. Ongoing evaluation is used to measure outcomes and adjust practices accordingly. When implementing intervention programs, the team:

	Desired Change/Goals	Barriers and Resources	Action Needed	Who	Priority/When
51. Targets communication goals primarily in an individual's natural environments during typical interactions, rather than in isolated environments.					
52. Uses pull-out intervention only when necessary for additional practice.	Establish criteria for when pull-out intervention should be used.	Staff time; consensus about when pull-out intervention is needed	Discuss criteria during team meetings.	Entire team	2	By beginning of next school year
53. Provides opportunities for initiation, maintenance, and termination of communication/ social interactions.					
54. Provides opportunities to communicate across all environments.					

C. Program Implementation

Program implementation is based on assessment and selected functional communication goals across settings. Ongoing evaluation is used to measure outcomes and adjust practices accordingly. When implementing intervention programs, the team:

	Desired Change/Goals	Barriers and Resources	Action Needed	Who	Priority/When
55. Uses an individual's current communication systems while promoting new skill acquisition.					
56. Uses communication supports and systems that are appropriate to each individual's physical abilities.					
57. Uses communication supports and systems that are appropriate to each individual's sensory abilities.	Work together to make sure all students who use AAC are supported, regardless of their cognitive abilities.	Some staff members believe students must have prerequisite skills before using AAC.	Provide current AAC literature, and discuss.	SLP / 1	By end of school year
58. Uses communication supports and systems that are appropriate to each individual's cognitive abilities.					

Example #2 / Action Plan Section II   CSC   197

C. Program Implementation

Program implementation is based on assessment and selected functional communication goals across settings. Ongoing evaluation is used to measure outcomes and adjust practices accordingly. When implementing intervention programs, the team:

	Desired Change/Goals	Barriers and Resources	Action Needed	Who	Priority/When
59. Uses communication supports and systems that are appropriate to an individual's communication needs and environments across settings.					
60. Includes necessary adaptations or modifications to the environment to optimize an individual's use of communication supports and systems (e.g., mounting AAC device on wheelchair).					
61. Provides for the seating and positioning needs of individuals who use communication supports and systems.	*Provide ergonomically supportive chairs for students who need them.*	*Funding*	*Review budget and priorities.*	*Entire team*	*3*	*At next budget review*
62. Makes assistive devices available to help individuals use supports for communication (e.g., hand/wrist splint, head-controlled pointer, control switches).					

C. Program Implementation

Program implementation is based on assessment and selected functional communication goals across settings. Ongoing evaluation is used to measure outcomes and adjust practices accordingly. When implementing intervention programs, the team:

	Desired Change/Goals	Barriers and Resources	Action Needed	Who	Priority/When
63. Integrates elements of individual instruction by all team members involved.	All team members should be encouraged to participate in intervention.	Sometimes team members wait for directions from teacher.	Discuss how each team member can contribute to intervention.	Whole team	2 Ongoing
64. Implements plans as designed to accomplish stated goals.					
65. Uses a team model that includes the individual, family members, friends, peers, professionals, support personnel, and other significant communication partners.					
66. Builds on goals and strategies developed in previous programs.					

C. Program Implementation

(continued)

Program implementation is based on assessment and selected functional communication goals across settings. Ongoing evaluation is used to measure outcomes and adjust practices accordingly. When implementing intervention programs, the team:	Desired Change/Goals	Barriers and Resources	Action Needed	Who	Priority/When
67. Includes and implements plans for continuity and transfer of information regarding communication supports and services before an individual changes program placement.					
68. Includes a specific time schedule for team reassessment of all program elements.					

Section III

Team Competencies

Example #2 / Action Plan Section III   CSC   201

A. Knowledge

CSC

Collectively, the team's knowledge supports and encourages communication. At least one team member has knowledge about:	Desired Change/Goals	Barriers and Resources	Action Needed	Who	Priority/When
69. Human development.					
70. Communication development, including reading and writing.	All team members will have _basic_ understanding of communication development.	In-service time & instructional resources	Propose training for spring in-service days; locate good resource people to provide this training.	SLPs	2 By early next spring
71. Individuals with severe disabilities across ages and levels of independence.					
72. Factors that prevent secondary conditions that interfere with communication (e.g., swallowing disorders, poor positioning, challenging behavior).					

A. Knowledge

Collectively, the team's knowledge supports and encourages communication. At least one team member has knowledge about:

	Desired Change/Goals	Barriers and Resources	Action Needed	Who	Priority/When
73. Different means of communication (e.g., body posture, vocalization, gaze, gesture, sign language, electronic and nonelectronic systems).					
74. Different types of communication symbols (e.g., pictures, braille, words, signs, speech).	All team members should understand basics about different types of symbols.	In-service time & instructional resources	Communication symbols will be addressed in in-service training along with communication development—see #70.	SLPs	2 / By early next spring
75. Amplification and other AT useful to people who have severe disabilities with accompanying sensory limitations.					
76. Medications and their effects on behavior, especially communication.					

Communication Supports Checklist • McCarthy et al. • © 1998 Paul H. Brookes Publishing Co., Inc., Baltimore

Example #2 / Action Plan Section III   CSC   203

A. Knowledge

(continued)

Collectively, the team's knowledge supports and encourages communication. At least one team member has knowledge about:	Desired Change/Goals	Barriers and Resources	Action Needed	Who	Priority/When
77. Motor control, muscle tone, and positioning as these affect communication.	At least one staff member who is present daily should have knowledge of motor control, muscle tone, & positioning.	Training for staff members	Identify appropriate workshop or short course, and submit request to administration.	SLPs	3 · Within 1 year
78. Disabilities that may co-occur with communication disorders (e.g., feeding and swallowing problems, seizures, sensory impairments).					
79. Challenging behavior as a potential communication act.					
80. Designing and working with a variety of service delivery models (e.g., classroom-based, pull-out, collaborative).					

Communication Supports Checklist • McCarthy et al. • © 1998 Paul H. Brookes Publishing Co., Inc., Baltimore

A. Knowledge

Collectively, the team's knowledge supports and encourages communication. At least one team member has knowledge about:

	Desired Change/Goals	Barriers and Resources	Action Needed	Who	Priority/When
81. Family dynamics and the impact of severe disability on the family.					
82. The importance of incorporating current research findings into assessment and program implementation.	AAC team members should keep up with new research related to AAC and communication supports.	Time (and motivation) to read professional journals after long day at work.	Form journal-sharing club to meet one evening every 2 months. Each person will report on one journal. Plan to go to dinner!	All SLPs	1 — Start *now*.

Communication Supports Checklist • McCarthy et al. • © 1998 Paul H. Brookes Publishing Co., Inc., Baltimore

Example #2 / Action Plan Section III   CSC   205

B. Skills and Experience

Team members' skills, experiences, and access to resources support and encourage communication. At least one team member has demonstrated the expertise or has the help of resource people who know how to:	Desired Change/Goals	Barriers and Resources	Action Needed	Who	Priority/When
83. Integrate the domains of cognitive, motor, sensory, and social functioning in communication *assessment* and *goal setting.*					
84. Integrate the domains of cognitive, motor, sensory, and social functioning in communication *implementation.*					
85. Provide ongoing assessment and evaluation using standardized and nonstandardized (formal or informal) procedures.	Develop simple, reliable system for assessing spontaneous communication in multiple settings.	We need a consultant to help us figure out how to do this.	Contact former professor, and see if she can refer a good consultant.	SLPs	2 By end of school year
86. Plan and implement communication assessments that lead directly to functional communication intervention goals and objectives.					

Communication Supports Checklist • McCarthy et al. • © 1998 Paul H. Brookes Publishing Co., Inc., Baltimore

B. Skills and Experience

(continued)

Team members' skills, experiences, and access to resources support and encourage communication. At least one team member has demonstrated the expertise or has the help of resource people who know how to:	Desired Change/Goals	Barriers and Resources	Action Needed	Who	Priority/When
87. Describe and document functional communication abilities and needs within specific contexts (e.g., educational settings, living environments, recreational environments, vocational environments, the community at large).	Team members should be able to describe students' communication in at least two settings outside of classroom.	1) Time for observation & support of staff 2) Form or checklist to record observations	1) Explain need to students, parents, principal, and other staff. 2) Develop checklist of things to observe/record.	SLPs, parents	2 — This spring
88. Plan, implement, monitor, and modify, as needed, intervention programs that allow individuals to develop functional communication skills in spoken or AAC modes appropriate to educational, living, recreational, and work environments.					
89. Assess emergent and functional literacy skills across all environments.					
90. Teach emergent and functional literacy skills across all environments.					

Communication Supports Checklist • McCarthy et al. • © 1998 Paul H. Brookes Publishing Co., Inc., Baltimore

Example #2 / Action Plan Section III   CSC   207

B. Skills and Experience

Team members' skills, experiences, and access to resources support and encourage communication. At least one team member has demonstrated the expertise or has the help of resource people who know how to:	Desired Change/Goals	Barriers and Resources	Action Needed	Who	Priority/When
91. Help the individual use the most appropriate (and least intrusive) positioning and mobility aids to maximize functional communication across a variety of environments.					
92. Manage activities of daily living and incorporate functional communication into each of these activities.	AAC staff and teachers will collaborate to integrate activities of daily living and functional communication.	Time to collaborate	Talk with principal about ways to do this.	SLPs and teachers	1 February
93. Integrate cognition; oral and written communication; and motor, sensory, and social development in defining and implementing communication goals.					
94. Incorporate current research findings into assessment and program implementation.					

B. Skills and Experience

Team members' skills, experiences, and access to resources support and encourage communication. At least one team member has demonstrated the expertise or has the help of resource people who know how to:

	Desired Change/Goals	Barriers and Resources	Action Needed	Who	Priority/When
95. Promote team participation and self-advocacy on the part of individuals with severe disabilities.	All team members should be able to promote participation and self-advocacy by students.	Lack of knowledge/experience; need in-service training on this subject	Request in-service training from staff development office.	SLPs	3 By end of next school year
96. Interact in a culturally sensitive manner.					
97. Understand laws that protect the rights of people with severe disabilities.					

Communication Supports Checklist • McCarthy et al. • © 1998 Paul H. Brookes Publishing Co., Inc., Baltimore

Example #2 / Action Plan Section III   CSC   209

Glossary

Assistive technology (AT)   Includes devices and services. An AT device is any item, piece of equipment, or product system, whether acquired commercially off the shelf, modified, or customized, that is used to increase, maintain, or improve functional capabilities of individuals with disabilities. An AT service is any service that directly assists an individual in selecting, obtaining, or using an AT device (Technology-Related Assistance for Individuals with Disabilities Act Amendments of 1994, PL 103-218).

Augmentative and alternative communication (AAC)   All forms of communication that enhance or supplement speech and writing. Different forms of AAC involve using communication boards, manual gestures or signs, and/or computers or other devices to communicate.

Challenging behavior   Challenging behavior is a behavior problem that may serve a communicative function. Examples of challenging behavior include shouting, hitting, crying, throwing objects, and head banging. For more information about providing communication supports to individuals with challenging behavior, see Mirenda (1997).

Communication supports   Clinical services, environmental modifications, assistive technology (AT), and guidance for communication partners that helps people with severe communication disabilities.

Communication symbol   A visual, auditory, and/or tactile representation of a conventional concept or object (e.g., gesture, photograph, manual sign, picto-ideograph, printed word, object, spoken word, braille). *See also* nonsymbolic communication, symbolic communication.

Communication systems   Communication modes and acts (e.g., intentional, nonintentional, high tech, low tech, gestural, spoken, written) that convey meaning.

Environmental goals   Goals that address desired changes in the practices or policies of an environment.

Individual goals   Goals that address desired changes for an individual's strengths, skills, communication, behavior, and so forth.

Intentional communication   Any act (motor or vocal, symbolic or nonsymbolic) that is intended to communicate one individual's meaning to another person.

Nonintentional communication   Any unconscious or involuntary act (motor or vocal, symbolic or nonsymbolic) that serves to communicate an individual's internal state or meaning to another person, even though the individual is not aware of the act and does not anticipate that it will have an effect on the other person.

Nonsymbolic communication   Communication in which the message is conveyed solely through direct physical action, indicative gestures, facial expression, and/or vocal intonation other than speech.

Person-centered planning   A method of life planning that includes the individual and centers around his or her desired goals, values, preferences, and areas of need. Formal approaches based on person-centered planning include Choosing Outcomes and Accommodations for Children (Giangreco, Cloninger, & Iverson, 1998), Making Action Plans (Lusthaus & Forest, 1987), Personal Futures Planning (Mount & Zwernik, 1988), and Planning Alternate Tomorrows with Hope (Pearpoint, O'Brien, & Forest, 1993).

Program   Organizational system that includes a variety of settings in which services are provided to individuals.

Pull-out intervention   Services or treatment delivered in settings removed from natural contexts.

Settings   All environments, places, or facilities within a program in which services are provided, including classrooms, gym classes, recreational settings, physical therapy rooms in rehabilitation centers, homes, and living areas in residential facilities.

Symbolic communication   Communication in which the message is conveyed through symbols that are distanced from the thing(s) they represent. Symbols vary along a continuum from very concrete symbols (e.g., a chain link that represents an outdoor swing) to completely arbitrary, abstract symbols (e.g., written words, spoken words).

REFERENCES

Giangreco, M.F., Cloninger, C.J., & Iverson, V.S. (1998). *Choosing outcomes and accommodations for children: A guide to educational planning for students with disabilities* (2nd ed.). Baltimore: Paul H. Brookes Publishing Co.

Lusthaus, E., & Forest, M. (1987). The kaleidoscope: A challenge to the cascade. In M. Forest (Ed.), *More education integration* (pp. 1–17). Downsview, Ontario, Canada: G. Allan Roeher Institute.

Mirenda, P. (1997). Supporting individuals with challenging behaviour through functional communication training and AAC: A research review. *Augmentative and Alternative Communication, 13,* 207–225.

Mount, B., & Zwernik, K. (1988). *It's never too early; it's never too late: A booklet about personal futures planning.* St. Paul, MN: Metropolitan Council.

Pearpoint, J., O'Brien, J., & Forest, M. (1993). *PATH.* Toronto, Ontario, Canada: Inclusion Press.

Technology-Related Assistance for Individuals with Disabilities Act Amendments of 1994, PL 103-218, 29 U.S.C. §§ 2201 *et seq.*